Milk A-Z

Robert Cohen

Argus Publishing
Englewood Cliffs, New Jersey

Published by Argus Publishing, 325 Sylvan Avenue, Englewood Cliffs, NJ 07632 (201-871-5871)

Printed in Canada

Cover Design and Illustrations by Brian Vigorita, Hopewell Junction, New York

ISBN # 0-9659196-8-4

To contact the author or the Dairy Education Board, please access the Internet: www.NOTMILK.com

A Note to the Reader

My goals are to provide you with information from peer-reviewed scientific journals and respected physicians, to overwhelm you with real science, and to shatter America's best marketed myth: Milk does the body good. During the next hour of absorbing knowledge from this book, you will find out that the exact opposite is true of the dairy industry's message.

After reading *A-Z*, I invite you to accept my challenge. Consume no milk or dairy products for just one week. No ice cream. No pizza. No cheese. Read labels. If you see "sodium caseinate" or "whey," say, "no way!"

If you are the typical American who eats 29.2 ounces per day of milk and dairy products (666 pounds per year), during your one-week experiment you should expel four quarts of mucous from your body. An internal "fog" will lift from your system. You'll sleep better, exercise better, have greater lung capacity, and you might even recapture your youth. You'll even be tempted to throw away your antacids, antihistamines, and other pills made unnecessary by your new discovery, NOTMILK!

On day eight, eat pizza for dinner and have ice cream for dessert, and your internal "sludge" will return in about twelve hours. That will be the most convincing moment of truth for you. My prediction: You'll forever give up all milk and dairy products.

This book cannot replace individualized medical care and advice from medical professionals. Find a healer who has taken courses in nutrition in medical school. Many physicians have not. Find an alternative practitioner who recognizes the age-old wisdom that you are what you eat.

I wish you the best of health.

A is for ALLERGIES

"Dairy products may play a major role in the development of allergies, asthma, sleep difficulties, and migraine headaches."

Pediatrics, 1989, 84(4)

"In reality, cow's milk, especially processed cow's milk, has been linked to a variety of health problems, including: mucous production, hemoglobin loss, childhood diabetes, heart disease, atherosclerosis, arthritis, kidney stones, mood swings, depression, irritability, and allergies."

Julie Klotter, M.D., Townsend Medical Letter, May, 1995

"At least 50% of all children in the United States are allergic to cow's milk, many undiagnosed. Dairy products are the leading cause of food allergy, often revealed by diarrhea, constipation, and fatigue. Many cases of asthma and sinus infections are reported to be relieved and even eliminated by cutting out dairy."

Nathaniel Mead, M.D., Natural Health, July, 1994

"Formula-fed babies, at the age of three months, were secreting low levels of serum antibodies to bovine proteins contained in their formula."

Pediatric-Allergy-Immunology, August, 1994, 5(3)

"Most formula-fed infants developed symptoms of allergic rejection to cow milk proteins before one month of age. About 50-70% experienced rashes or other skin symptoms, 50-60 percent gastrointestinal symptoms, and 20-30 percent respiratory symptoms. The recommended therapy is to avoid cow's milk."

Pediatric-Allergy-Immunology, August, 1994, 5(5 Supplement)

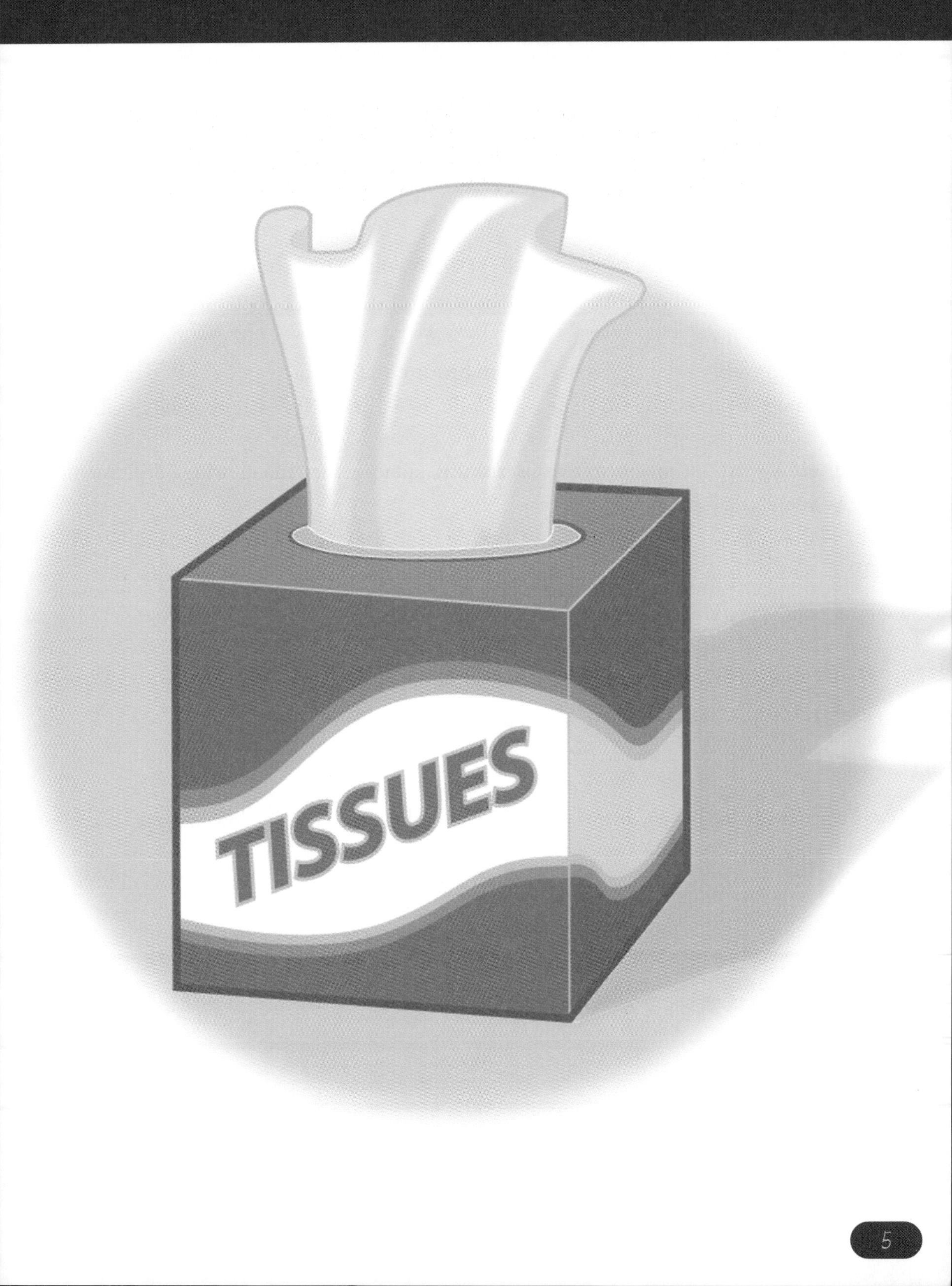
TISSUES

B is for BREAST CANCER

There are hundreds of millions of different proteins in nature, and only one hormone that is identical between any two species. That powerful growth hormone is insulin-like growth factor, or IGF-I. IGF-I survives digestion and has been identified as the KEY FACTOR in breast cancer's growth. IGF-I is identical in human and cow. By drinking cow's milk, one delivers IGF-I to the body's cells.

"Human insulin-like growth factor (IGF-I) and bovine IGF-I are identical."
Science, vol. 249, August 24, 1990

"IGF-I is critically involved in the aberrant growth of human breast cancer cells."
Journal of the National Institutes of Health, 1991, 3

"Estrogen regulation of IGF-I in breast cancer cells would support the hypothesis that IGF-I has a regulatory function in breast cancer."
Molecular Cell Endocrinology, March, 99(2)

"IGF-I is a potent growth factor for cellular proliferation in the human breast carcinoma cell line."
Journal of Cellular Physiology, January, 1994, 158(1)

"IGF-I plays a major role in breast cancer cell growth."
European Journal of Cancer, 29A (16), 1993

"IGF-I produces a 10-fold increase in RNA levels of cancer cells. IGF-I appears to be a critical component in cellular proliferation."
Experimental Cell Research, March, 1994, 211(1)

"Serum IGF-I levels increased significantly in milk drinkers, an increase of about 10% above baseline but was unchanged in the control group."

Journal of the American Dietetic Association, vol. 99, no. 10, October 1999

"IGF-I accelerates the growth of breast cancer cells."

Science, Vol. 259, January 29, 1993

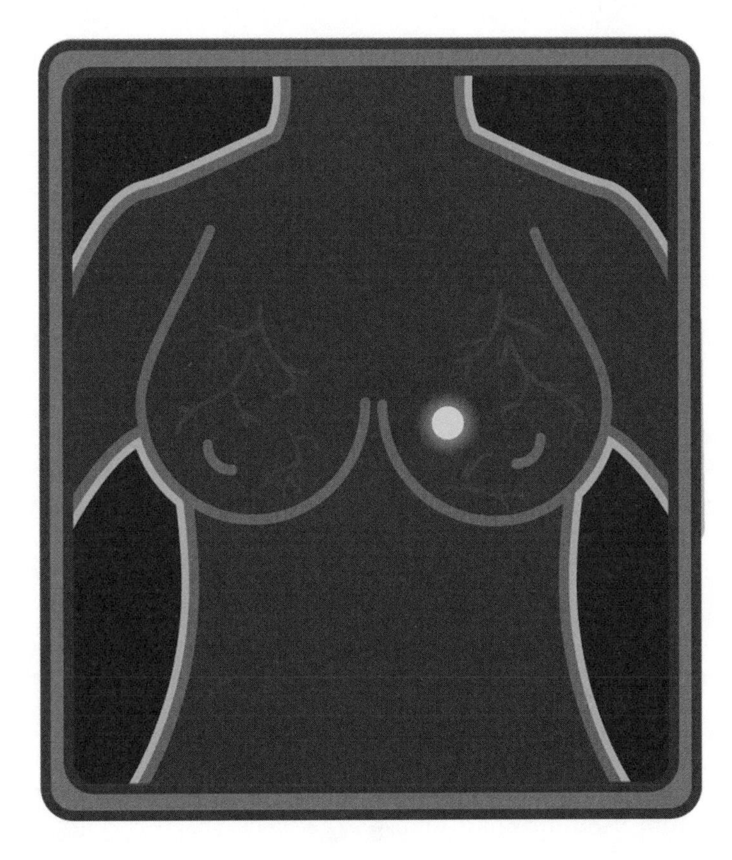

C is for CROHN'S DISEASE

The most serious of bacterial cow diseases for American dairymen is caused by mycobacterium paratuberculosis. This bacterium causes a bovine disease called "Johne's." Cows diagnosed with Johne's Disease have diarrhea and heavy fecal shedding of bacteria. These bacteria become cultured in milk, and are not destroyed by pasteurization. Occasionally, the milkborne bacteria will begin to grow in the human host, and irritable bowel syndrome and Crohn's results.

"It is reasonable to conjecture that M. paratuberculosis may be responsible for some cases of Crohn's disease."

Journal of Clinical Microbiology, 1992; 30(12)

"Johne's disease and Crohn's disease are remarkably similar in clinical signs and intestinal pathology."

Hoard's Dairyman, January 24, 1995

"Of 77 milk samples (from cows with Johne's disease), 11.6% were culture-positive (contained M. paratubercolosis)."

Journal of Clinical Microbiology, 1992; 30(1)

"Mycobacterium paratuberculosis was isolated from tissue taken from patients with Crohn's disease and is implicated in the etiology of this disease."

Journal of Clinical Microbiology, 1993, May 31(5)

"Mycobacterium Paratuberculosis crosses the species barrier to infect and cause disease in humans."

British Medical Journal, Feb 1998, 315

"Mycobacterium paratuberculosis is capable of surviving commercial pasteurization, when there are more than 10 bacteria per milliliter in raw milk."

Applied and Environmental Microbiology: 64(3), March 1998

"Mycobacterium paratuberculosis RNA was found in 100% of Crohn's disease patients, compared with 0% of controls."

Proceedings National Academy of Sciences USA : 93: September, 1996

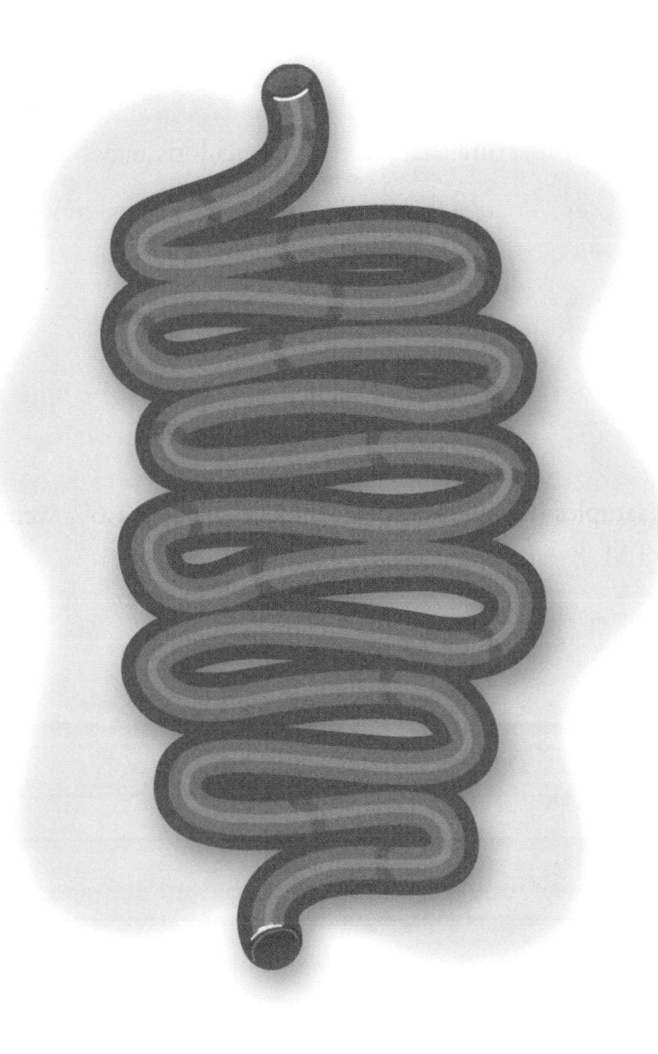

D is for DIABETES

"Studies have suggested that bovine serum albumin is the milk protein responsible for the onset of diabetes...Patients with insulin-dependent diabetes mellitus produce antibodies to cow milk proteins that participate in the development of islet dysfunction...Taken as a whole, our findings suggest that an active response in patients with IDDM (to the bovine protein) is a feature of the autoimmune response."

New England Journal of Medicine, July 30, 1992

"The National Dairy Board's slogan, 'Milk. It does a body good,' sounds a little hollow these days."

Scientific American, October, 1992

"In lieu of the recent evidence that cow's milk protein may be implicated in the pathogenesis of diabetes mellitus, we believe that the Committee on Nutrition should clarify whether cow's milk is ever appropriate for children and whether or not infant formulas that are based on cow's milk protein are appropriate alternatives to breast milk."

Pediatrics, July, 1992: 89

"Antibodies to bovine beta-casein are present in over a third of IDDM patients and relatively non-existent in healthy individuals."

The Lancet, October, 1996, 348

"Introduction of dairy products and high milk consumption during childhood may increase the child's risk of developing juvenile diabetes."

Diabetologia, 1994; 37(4)

"The first pilot stage of our IDD prevention study found that oral exposure to dairy milk proteins in infancy resulted in both cellular and immune response... this suggests the possible importance of the immune system to the pathogenesis of IDD."

The Lancet, Dec 14, 1996

"These new studies, and more than 20 well-documented previous ones, have prompted one researcher to say the link between milk and juvenile diabetes is 'very solid.'"

Diabetes Care 1994, 17 (12)

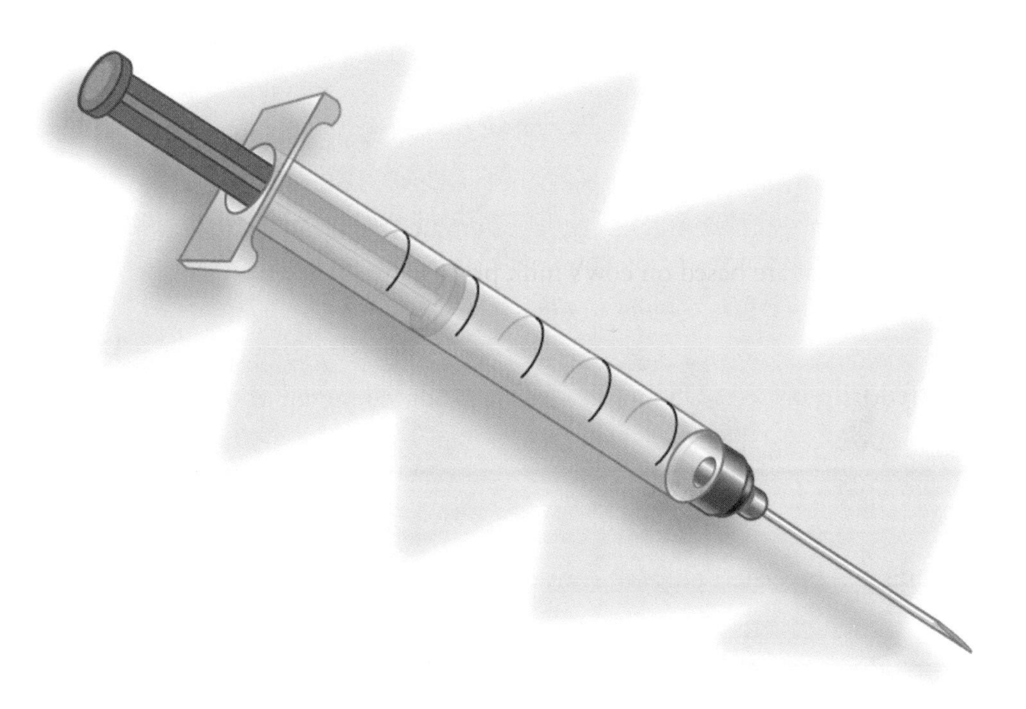

E is for EAR INFECTIONS

"Milk allergies are very common in children...They are the leading cause of the chronic ear infections that plague up to 40% of all children under the age of six."

Julian Whitaker, M.D., Health & Healing, October, 1998, Volume 8, No. 10

"Cow's milk allergy is associated with recurrent otitis media (ear infection) during childhood."

Acta Otolaryngol 1999; 119(8)

"If a bottlefed baby has an ear infection, eliminate milk and dairy products from the child's diet for thirty days to see if any benefits result...a cause of frequent ear infections in children is food allergies."

James Balch, M.D., Prescription for Nutritional Healing

"Concerning ear infections, you just don't see this painful condition among infants and children who aren't getting cow's milk into their systems."

William Northrup, M.D., Natural Health July, 94

"Breastfeeding protects US infants against the development of diarrhea and ear infection."

Pediatrics, June, 1997: 99(6)

"Cow's milk has become a point of controversy among doctors and nutritionists. There was a time when it was considered very desirable, but research has forced us to rethink this recommendation...dairy products contribute to a surprising number of health problems (including) chronic ear problems..."

Benjamin Spock, M.D., Child Care, 7th Edition

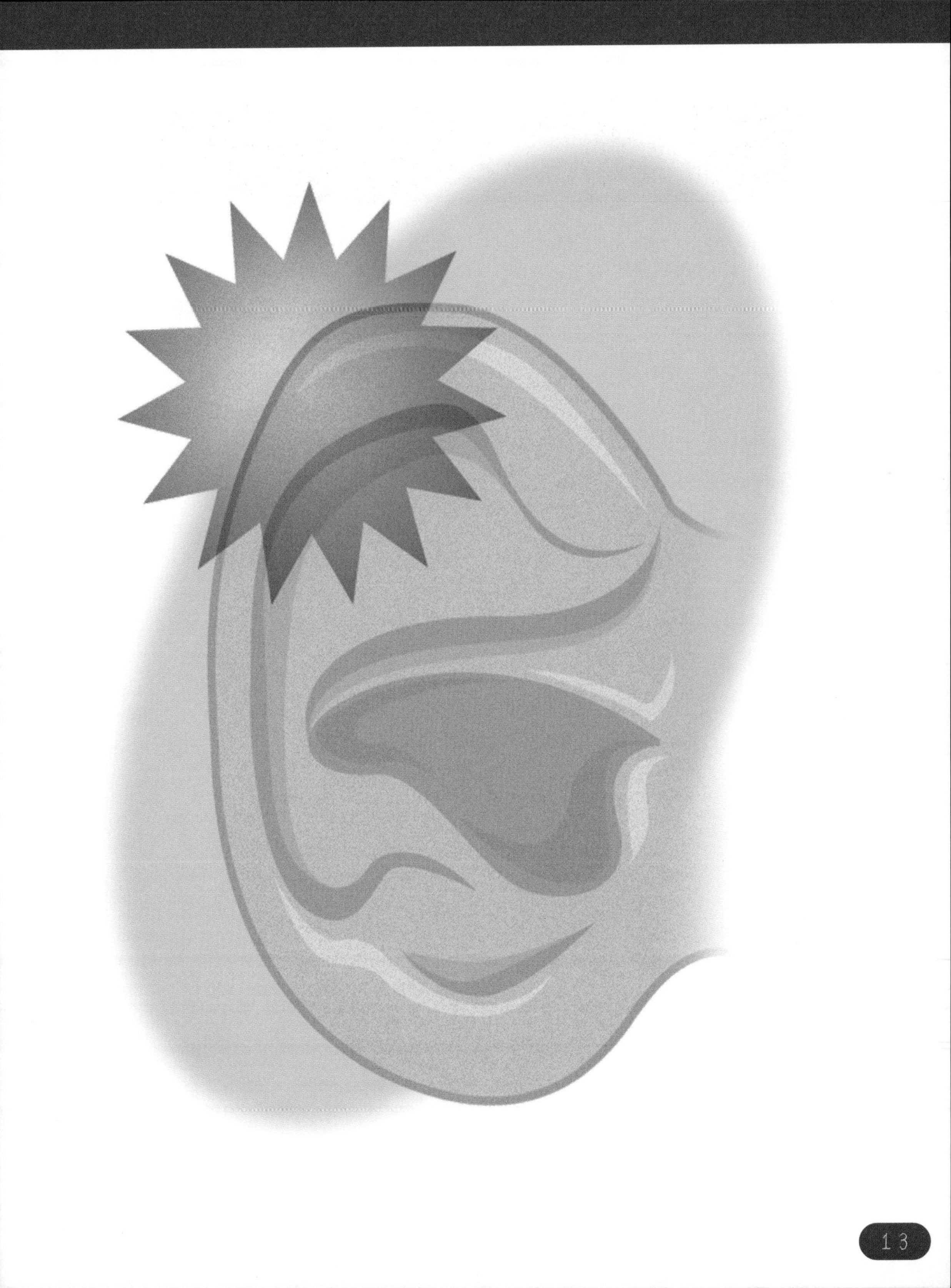

F is for FAT

"The most popular definition for fat is a 'greasy or oily substance.' Milk fat and the associated lipid material are present in milk...about 1500 billion or more may be found in a pint of milk. The fats of plant origin in the cow's diet contain large amounts of polyunsaturated fatty acids. These fats are hydrolyzed in the cow's rumen. The liberated fatty acids are then converted into saturated fatty acids."

Lincoln Lampert, Modern Dairy Products, Third Edition

"From 1965 to 1996, a considerable shift in the adolescent diet occurred... increases occurred in the consumption of higher fat potatoes and mixed dishes (pizza, macaroni & cheese)...These trends, far greater than for US adults, may compromise the health of the future US population."

Archives of Disabled Child, 2000 Jul, 83:1

"Dietary fat during childhood may be more life-threatening than was originally suspected... Overweight children are usually the victims of the dietary habits of the adult members of the family...Reducing dietary fat to levels necessary to the control of cholesterol cannot be achieved if a child drinks whole milk or eats cheese."

Charles Attwood, M.D., Dr. Attwood's Low-Fat Prescription for Kids

"Milk fat has been identified as a cholesterol-elevating fat because it contains cholesterol and is primarily saturated."

Journal of Dairy Science, 1991; 74 (11)

"Preference for a diet high in animal fat could be a pathogenic factor, and milk and high fat dairy products contribute considerably to dietary fat intake."

Journal of the American College of Nutrition, 2000 Apr, 19:2 Supplement

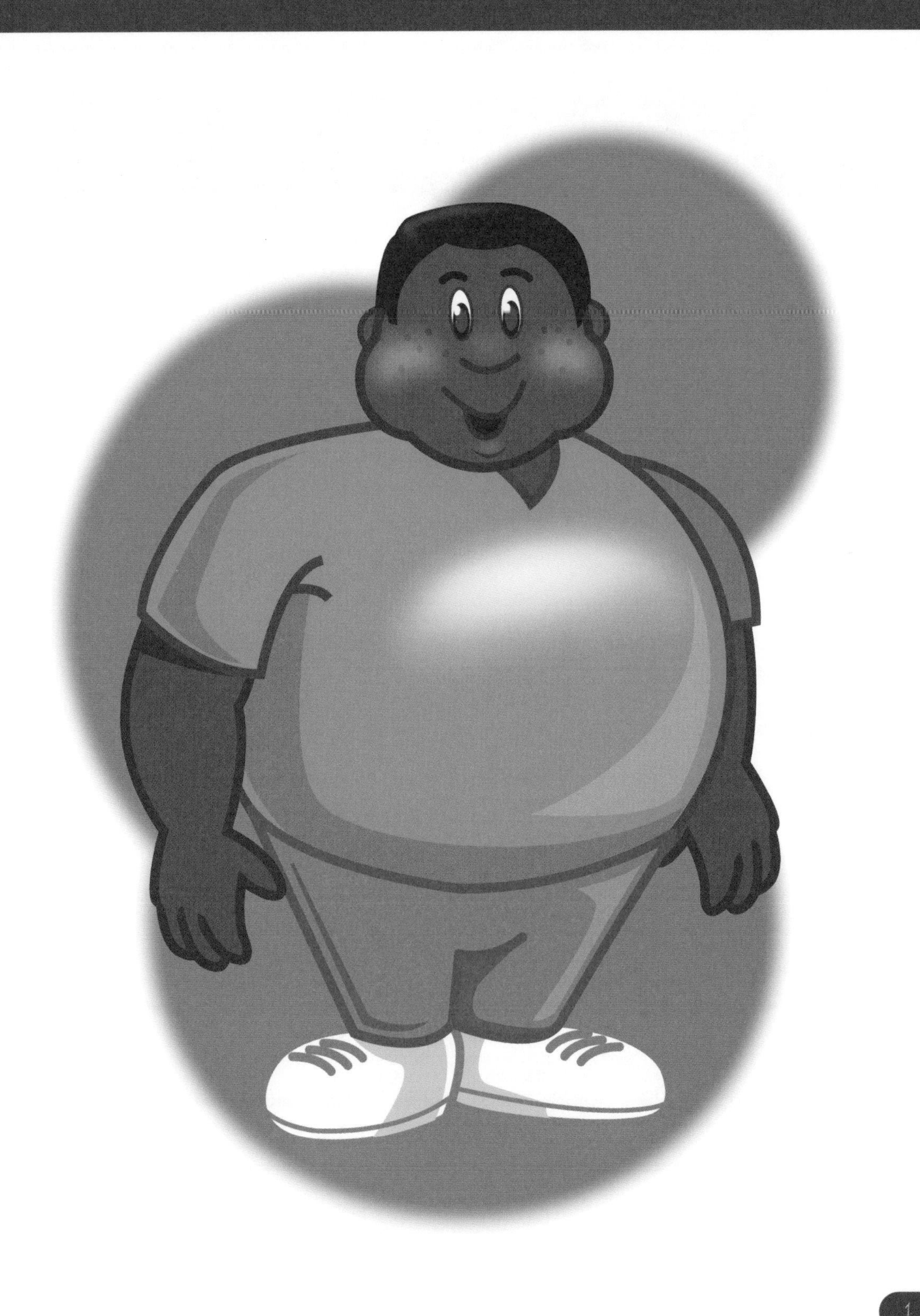

G is for GROWTH HORMONES

Insulin-like growth factor (IGF-I) in humans and cows are identical. Like a key fitting into a lock, this hormone is a perfect match between two species of animal, and exerts powerful growth effects. IGF-I is the most powerful growth hormone in the human body. Every sip of milk and every bite of cheese contains IGF-I.

"BGH-treated milk is safe because it is indistinguishable from normal milk."

Executive Branch Report on rbGH, February 9, 1994

"Recombinant rbGH treatment produces an increase in the concentration of insulin-like growth factor-I (IGF-I) in cow's milk."

FDA review of genetically engineered milk, Science, Vol. 249, 8/24/90

"A strong positive association was observed between IGF-I levels and prostate cancer risk."

Science, vol. 279, January 23, 1998

"Insulin-like growth factor (IGF)-I, a mitogenic and antiapoptotic peptide, can affect the proliferation of breast epithelial cells, and is thought to have a role in breast cancer."

The Lancet, vol. 351, May 9, 1998

"Insulin-like growth factor-I (IGF-I) is expressed in many tumor cell lines and has a role in both normal cell proliferation and in the growth of cancers."

Cancer Gene Therapies, 2000 Mar, 7:3

"Insulin-like growth factors (IGFs), in particular IGF-I and IGF-II, strongly stimulate the proliferation of a variety of cancer cells, including those from lung cancer."

Journal of the National Cancer Institute, vol. 91, no. 2., January 20, 1999

"The insulin-like growth factor (IGF) system is widely involved in human carcinogenesis. A significant association between high circulating IGF-I concentrations and an increased risk of lung, colon, prostate and pre-menopausal breast cancer has recently been reported."

International Journal of Cancer, 2000 Aug, 87:4

"Serum IGF-I levels increased significantly in the milk drinking group…an increase of about 10% above baseline-but was unchanged in the control group."

Journal of the American Dietetic Association, vol. 99, no. 10. October 1999

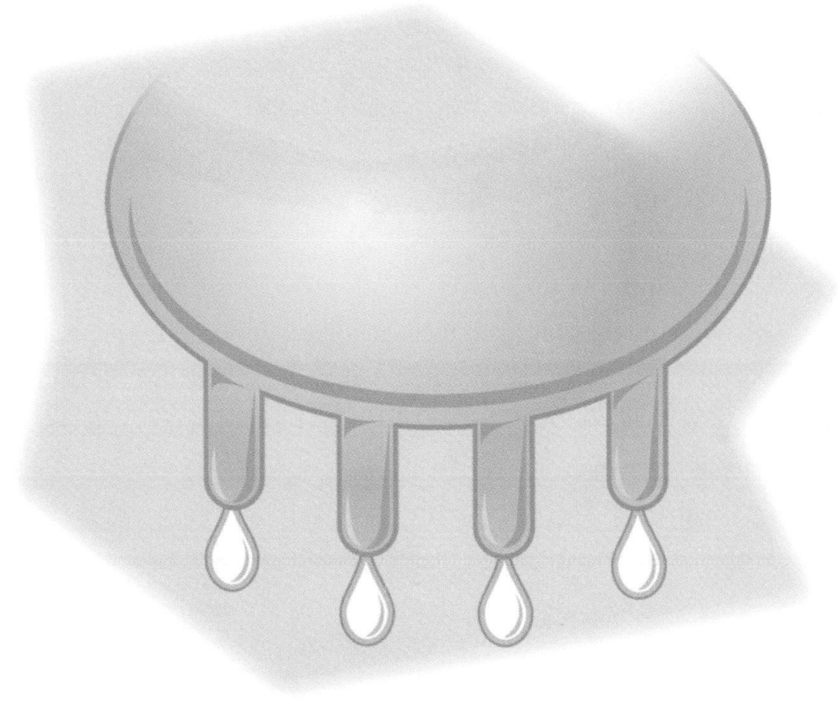

H is for HEART DISEASE

Heart disease is America's number one killer. Most Americans and scientific agencies are in agreement: Saturated animal fat and cholesterol do not do the heart any good. According to USDA figures, each day, the average American eats just 5 ounces of meat and chicken containing saturated fat and cholesterol, and 29.2 ounces of milk and dairy products (666 pounds per American) containing the same dangerous factors.

"Milk and milk products gave the highest correlation coefficient to heart disease, while sugar, animal proteins and animal fats came in second, third, and fourth, respectively."

Survey of Mortality Rates and Food Consumption Statistics of 24 Countries, Medical Hypothesis, 7:907-918, 1981

"More patients who had suffered a myocardial infarction had elevated levels of antibodies against milk proteins than was found in a comparable group of patients without coronary heart disease."

The Lancet, ii: 205-207, 1980

"Excessive milk consumption may adversely affect the circulation on account of the high calcium content of milk and because lactose promotes the intestinal absorption of calcium. Excessive calcium intake may cause calcification and rigidification of the large elastic arteries, which could be an important factor in causing myocardial ischaemia."

Medical Hypotheses, 2000 May, 54:5

"Milk consumption correlates positively with cholesterol levels in blood as well as coronary mortality. In comparisons between 17 countries, there is a good correlation between national cholesterol levels and mortality from ischemic heart disease."

European Journal of Clinical Nutrition, 48, 1994

"Milk and many components of milk (butterfat, milk protein, calcium from milk, and riboflavin)...were positively related to coronary heart disease mortality for all 40 countries studied."

Circulation, 1993; 88(6)

"For ischemic heart disease milk carbohydrates were found to have the highest statistical association for males aged 35+ and females aged 65+."

Alternative Medical Review, 1998 Aug, 3:4

I is for IRON DEFICIENCY

Millions of Americans suffer from a hidden disease called anemia. The most common cause of anemia is iron deficiency. Red blood cells have a life of about four months, and lack of iron leads to an inability to manufacture new cells. Hundreds of ailments can result from too-little iron, and milk consumption has been shown to cause intestinal bleeding, resulting in low hemoglobin count. The result: weakness, depression, irritability.

"Cow's milk can cause blood loss from the intestinal tract, which over time, reduces the body's iron stores. Blood loss may be a reaction to cow's milk proteins."

Journal of Pediatrics, 1990, 116

"Babies who are fed whole cow's milk during the second six months of life may experience a 30% increase in intestinal blood loss and a significant loss of iron in their stools."

Pediatrics, 1982; 89(6)

"Children with iron deficiency had a higher intake of cow's milk compared to those with sufficient iron. Intake of cow's milk is significantly higher in children with iron deficiency."

Acta Paediatrica, 1999 Dec, 88:12

"Cow's milk-induced intestinal bleeding is a well-recognized cause of rectal bleeding in infancy. In all cases, bleeding resolved completely after instituting a cow's milk-free diet."

Journal of Pediatric Surgery, 1999 Oct, 34:10

"Infants who consume cow's milk during infancy are at increased risk of anemia. Breast milk is the ideal."

Public Health Nutrition, 1998 Jun, 1:2

"Cow's milk allergy (CMA) is one of the most common food allergies in young infants...The clinical presentation of these infants may be very traumatic to their parents, as significant rectal bleeding is the most common symptom in this disease."

West Virginia Medical Journal, 1999 Sep-Oct; 95(5)

"In reality, cow's milk, especially processed cow's milk, has been linked to a variety of health problems, including hemoglobin loss, mood swings, depression, and irritability."

Townsend Medical Letter, May, 1995

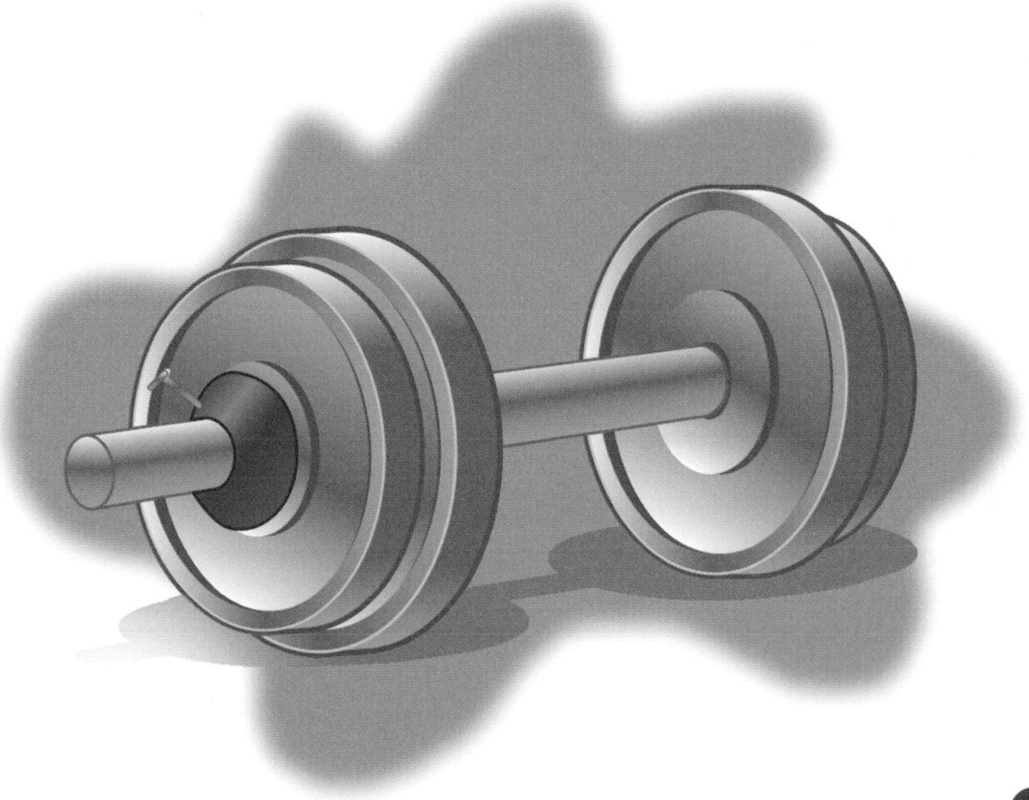

J is for JUVENILE ILLNESSES

"At least 50% of all children in the United States are allergic to milk, many undiagnosed. Dairy products are the leading cause of food allergy, often revealed by constipation, diarrhea, and fatigue. Many cases of asthma and sinus infections are reported to be relieved and even eliminated by cutting out dairy."

Frank Oski, M.D., Chief of Pediatrics at Johns Hopkins Medical School
Don't Drink Your Milk, July, 1994

"Chronic diarrhea is the most common gastrointestinal symptom of intolerance of cow's milk among children...cow's milk can also cause severe perianal lesions with pain on defecation and consequent constipation in young children. In young children, chronic constipation can be a manifestation of intolerance of cow's milk."

New England Journal of Medicine, 1998 Oct, 339:16

"Allergic asthma and rhinitis, atopic dermatitis (AD), urticaria and gastrointestinal allergy, are common diseases of infants and children. Cow's milk appears to be the most common offending food both in gastrointestinal and in cutaneous manifestations of atopic disease. It was recently estimated that 14% of children suffer from AD and about 25% from adverse reactions to cow's milk."

European Review Medical Pharmacological Science, 1998 May

"Cow's milk allergy is a disease of infancy and usually appears in the first few months of life. The evaluation of infants for possible cow's milk allergy is one of the more common problems encountered by pediatricians."

European Science Medical Farmacologia, 1990 Aug, 12(4-5)

"Cow's milk allergy (CMA) is a common disease of infancy and childhood. An appropriate cow's milk substitute is necessary for feeding babies with CMA."

Journal of Allergy & Clinical Immunology, 1999 Jun, 103:6

K is for KILLER BACTERIA

By the time one hears the snap, crackle, and pop from a bowl of Rice Krispies, that milk has been pasteurized three times. Another secret the dairy industry does not want you to know. Why doesn't the first time work, or the second, or third? Most people have experienced the putrid smell of soured milk. Pour it down the drain on day eight. Imagine what you consumed on day seven?

"A drop of sour milk may contain more than 50 million bacteria...certain bacteria, especially organisms belonging to the genera bacillus and clostridium, have the ability to transform themselves into small bodies called spores. The word spore comes from the Greek word for seed. The spore can often withstand drying, the temperature of boiling water (pasteurization), and the action of some germicides. When suitable conditions return, the spore resumes its vegetative form and the bacterium again returns to the usual activities of its normal life cycle."

Lincoln Lampert, Modern Dairy Products, Third Edition

"Milk from cows inoculated with listeria was pooled for 2 to 4 days and then heated at 162 degrees Fahrenheit for 16 seconds in a high-temperature, short-time pasteurization unit. Live listeria bacteria was then successfully isolated from the milk after heat treatment in 11 of 12 pasteurization trials."

Journal of Environmental Microbiology, July 1987 (53)

"Salmonella can remain viable in butter for up to 9 months."

Journal of Dairy Science 1992; 75 (9):2339

"Listeria organisms excreted in cow's milk escaped pasteurization, grew well at refrigerator temperatures, and were ingested by consumers."

New England Journal of Medicine, 1985, 312 (7)

"Bulk tank milk from 131 dairy herds in eastern South Dakota and western Minnesota were examined for coliforms and noncoliform bacteria. Coliforms were detected in 62.3% of bulk tank milk samples...noncoliform bacteria were observed in 76.3% of bulk tank milk."

Journal of Dairy Science, 1999 Dec, 82:12

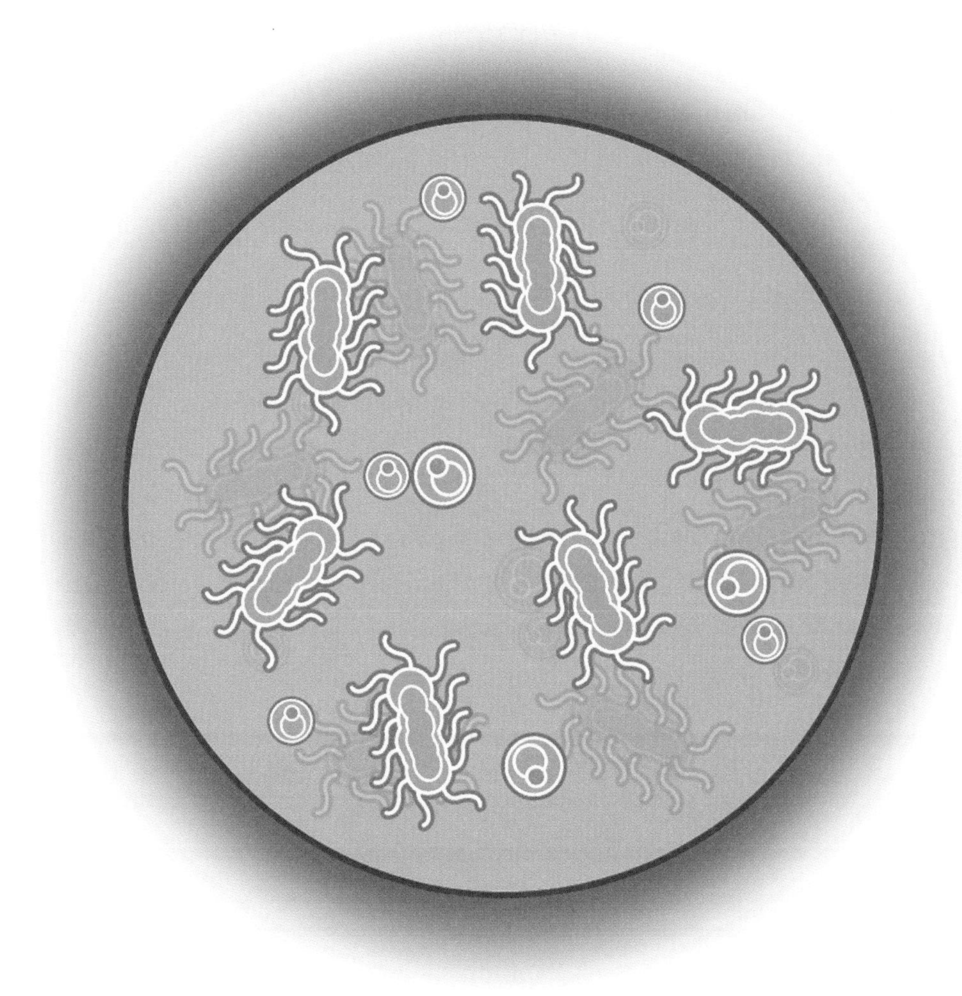

L is for LACTOSE INTOLERANCE

Lactose, a milk sugar, is made up of two sugars, glucose and galactose. Most adults "lack" the enzyme, lactase, to break down lactose. Instead, lactose is broken down by bacteria in the lower intestines. Bacteria eat too. Problem is, after bacteria dine, their own body wastes combine with those sugars to ferment into gas and toxins, causing bloating and cramps.

"An estimated 50 million Americans experience intestinal discomfort after consuming dairy products. Symptoms include bloating, stomach pain, cramps, gas, or diarrhea."

Postgraduate Medicine, 1994; 95(1)

"Human adult-onset lactase decline is a biologic feature characteristic of the maturing intestine in the majority of the world's population."

Nutritional Review, 1998 Jan, 56:1 Pt 1

"Lactose intolerance is widespread...Lactose maldigestion may coexist in adults with irritable bowel syndrome and in children with recurrent abdominal pain. Management consists primarily of dietary changes."

Postgraduate Medical Journal, 1998 Sep, 104:3

"Overall, about 75 percent of the world's population, including 25 percent of those in the U.S., lose their lactase enzymes after weaning."

Journal of the American Dietetic Association, 1996; 9

"Lactose malabsorption and lactase deficiency are chronic organic pathologic conditions characterized by abdominal pain and distention, flatulence, and the passage of loose, watery stools…introduction of a lactose-free dietary regime relieves symptoms in most patients who remain largely unaware of the relationship between food intake and symptoms."

Journal of Clinical Gastroenterology, 1999 Apr, 28:3

"Females with lactose malabsorption not only showed signs of irritable bowel syndrome but also signs of premenstrual syndrome and mental depression... Lactose malabsorption should be considered in patients with signs of mental depression."

Digestive Science, 1998 Nov, 43:11

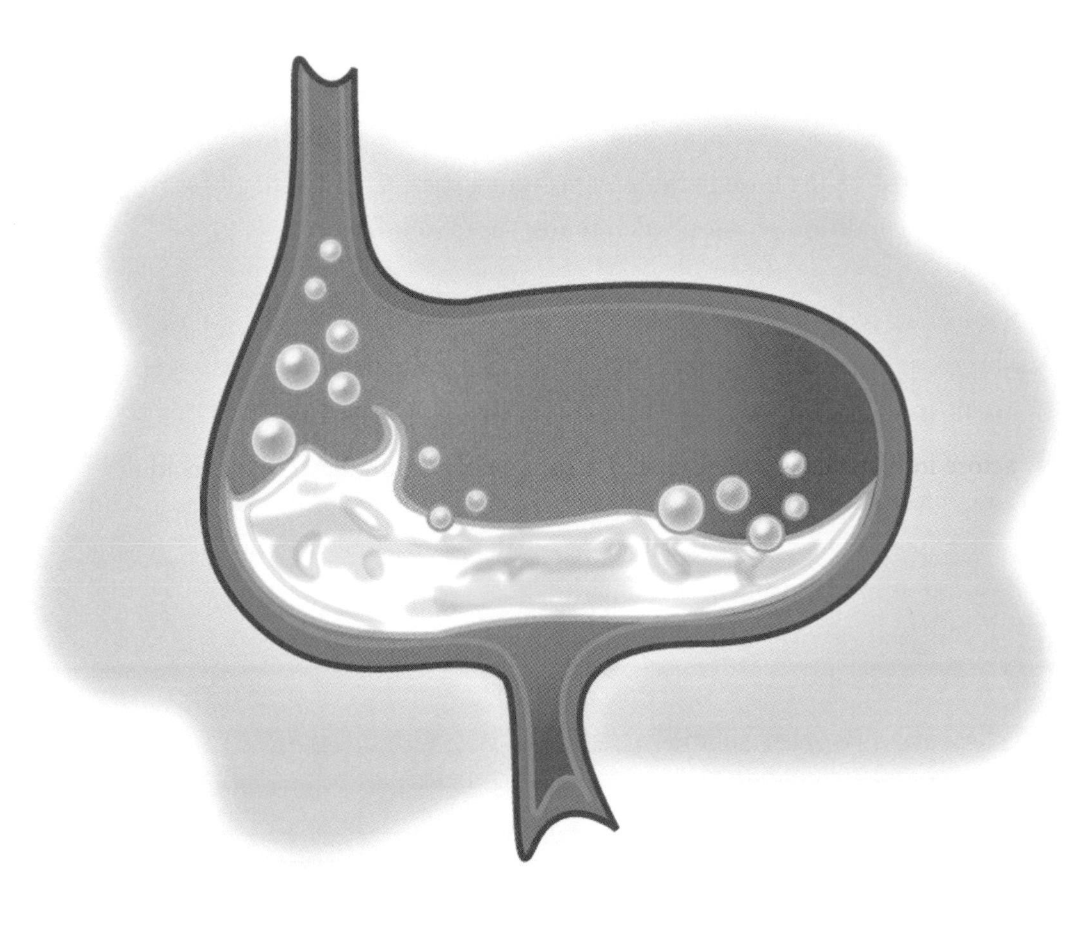

M is for MAD COW DISEASE

In 1907, Dr. Alzheimer published a treatise about a disease that would one day carry his name. He had two young colleagues who worked with him, Dr. Creutzfeldt and Dr. Jakob, and they too identified a similar brain-wasting disease that now has Europe in a panic. The brains of cows turn into a sponge-like mass and their behavior is called "mad." The human variant of Mad Cow Disease has been named Creutzfeldt Jakob Disease, or CJD. The protein causing CJD has no DNA, and has been described as more like a crystal than cellular material. In labs, 1000 degree Fahrenheit heat does not destroy this protein particle. Some scientists say that once infected, the incubation period can last anywhere from one month to thirty years. As the human brain turns into a sponge, this spongioform encephalitic condition physically debilitates those so infected.

"Compelling scientific evidence suggests so-called prion disease can and has infected humans...at present, there is no reliable antemortem diagnosis, specific treatment, or vaccine to prevent the disease. The agent thought to be responsible for this unusual class of disease is a rogue protein (called a prion) that, unlike all other agents known to cause infectious disease, contains neither DNA nor RNA. The "bad" prion forms holes or a spongy appearance in the brain in all disease variants, hence the generic designation of spongiform encephalopathy."

Quintessence International, 1998 May, 29:5

"A 24-year-old vegetarian has been diagnosed with Cruetzfeld-Jacob disease. Scientists fear that milk and cheese may be the source of infection."

Michael Hornsby, London Times, August 23, 1997

"The destruction of milk from suspected cows was recommended in England to insure the public's safety...Experiments also indicate that temperatures reached during pasteurization of milk and household cooking does not kill the agent. In the United Kingdom on December 1, 1988 the government announced a ban on the sale of milk from infected cattle..."

Virgil Hulse, M.D., Mad Cows and Milkgate

"Transmission of prions from infected cattle to humans by oral intake seems not only possible but also very probable."

Annals of Italian Medicine, 1998 Oct, 13:4

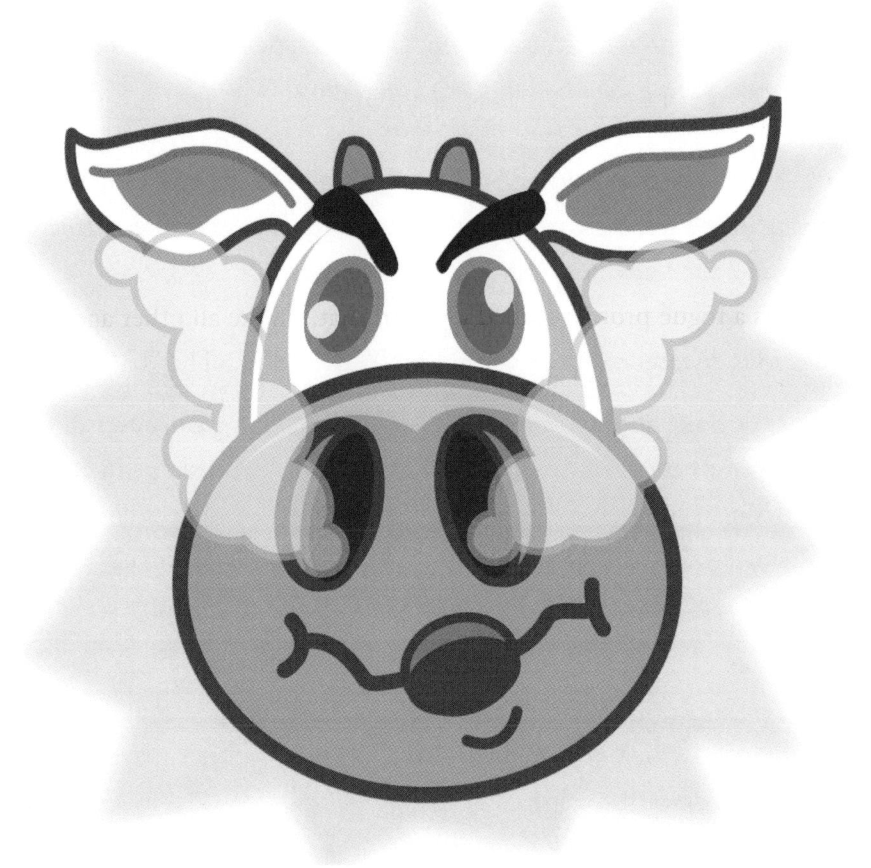

N is for NASAL CONGESTION

Long distance runners know. Opera singers know. Broadway actors and actresses are told not to consume milk or dairy products or their voices will become "phlegmy." Eighty percent of milk protein is casein, a tenacious glue and allergenic protein. Eat casein and you produce histamines, then mucous. The reaction is often delayed, occurring 12-15 hours after consumption. Few people note the ill effects because milk and dairy products represent 40% of what the average American eats (about 666 pounds per American per year), and these proteins are continuously eaten. By eliminating ALL milk and dairy for just one week, most people note the differences, which include better sleep, more energy, better bowel movements, clarity in thought, muscle, bone, and back pain relief. Oh, yes. NOTMILK means saying goodbye to nasal congestion.

"Sixty-two percent of the children were confirmed to be allergic to milk..." (153 hospitalized infants with pneumonia or bronchitis were tested)

Roczniki Akademii Medycznej, 1995; 40(3) (Polish journal)

"Cow's milk protein often persists beyond 4 years of age. Clinical presentation changed over time: at onset symptoms were prevalently gastrointestinal, while at the end of the study there was an increased frequency of wheezing and constipation and a higher frequency of delayed reactions...infants with persistent cow's milk protein intolerance exhibited atopic disease: asthma, rhinitis, eczema."

Journal of Clinical Experimental Allergy, 1998 Jul, 28:7

"Symptoms seen most frequently in babies who are identified as allergic to cow's milk included diarrhea, repeated vomiting, eczema, recurrent attacks of nasal congestion, and recurrent bronchitis."

Frank Oski, M.D., Don't Drink Your Milk

"Some textbooks of pediatrics either avoid mentioning cow's milk allergy or only lightly refer to it...On the other hand, there are those, particularly among pediatricians, and to a lesser extent among general practitioners, who over-zealously label infants 'milk sensitive' and who are inclined to recommend discontinuing the use of cow's milk whenever an infant has a gastrointestinal upset, respiratory symptom, or a skin rash."

SL Bahna, M.D., DC Heiner, M.D., Allergies to Milk

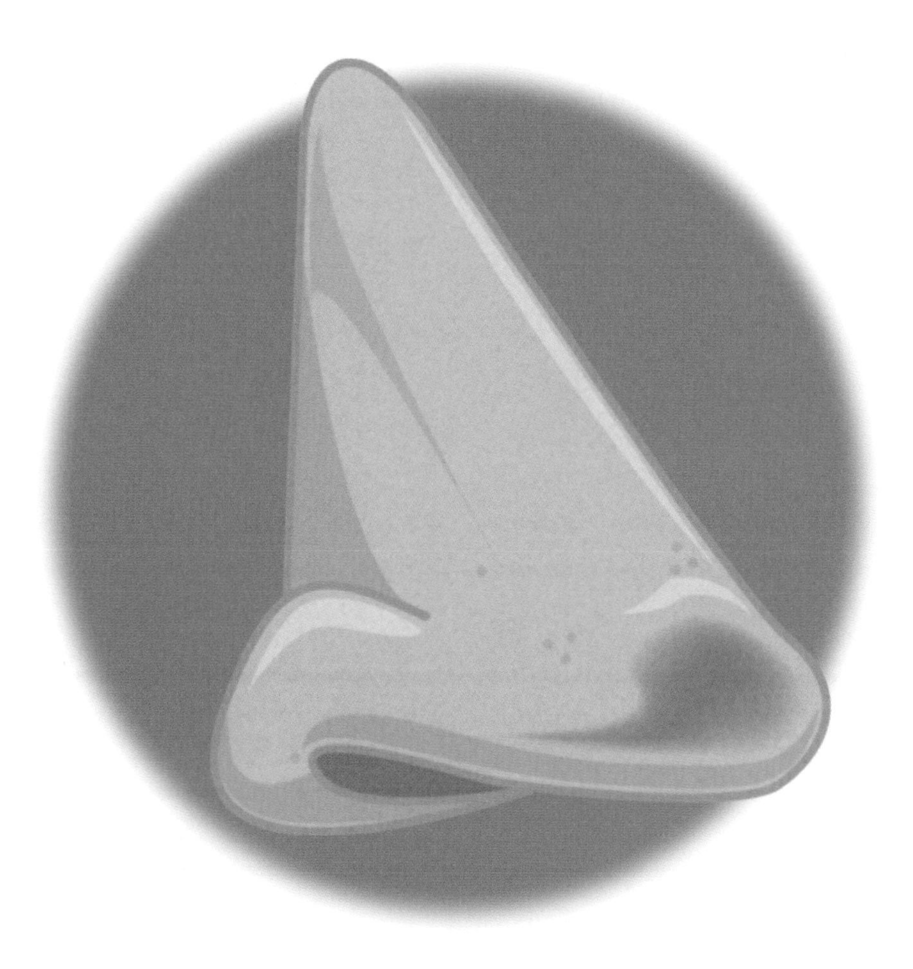

O is for OSTEOPOROSIS

American women have been consuming an average of two pounds of milk per day for their entire lives, yet thirty million American women have osteoporosis. Drinking milk does not prevent bone loss. Bone loss is accelerated by ingesting more protein than the body requires. Milk has been called "liquid meat." In order to absorb calcium, the body needs comparable amounts of magnesium. Milk and dairy products contain only small amounts of magnesium. Magnesium is the center atom of chlorophyll.

"Osteoporosis is caused by a number of things, one of the most important being too much dietary protein."

Science, 1986; 233

"Increasing one's protein intake by 100% may cause calcium loss to double."

Journal of Nutrition, 1981; 111 (3)

"Even when eating 1,400 mg of calcium daily, one can lose up to 4% of his or her bone mass each year while consuming a high-protein diet."

American Journal of Clinical Nutrition, 1979; 32(4)

"Calcium intake demonstrated no protective in preventing bone fractures. In fact, those populations with the highest calcium intakes had higher fracture rates than those with more modest calcium intakes."

California Tissue International, 1992; 50

"Countries with the highest rates of osteoporosis, such as the U.S., England, and Sweden, consume the most milk."

Nutrition Action Healthletter, June, 1993

"There is no significant association between teenaged milk consumption and the risk of adult fractures...women consuming greater amounts of calcium from dairy foods had significantly increased risks of hip fractures."

Harvard study of 78,000 women, American Journal of Public Health, 1997;87

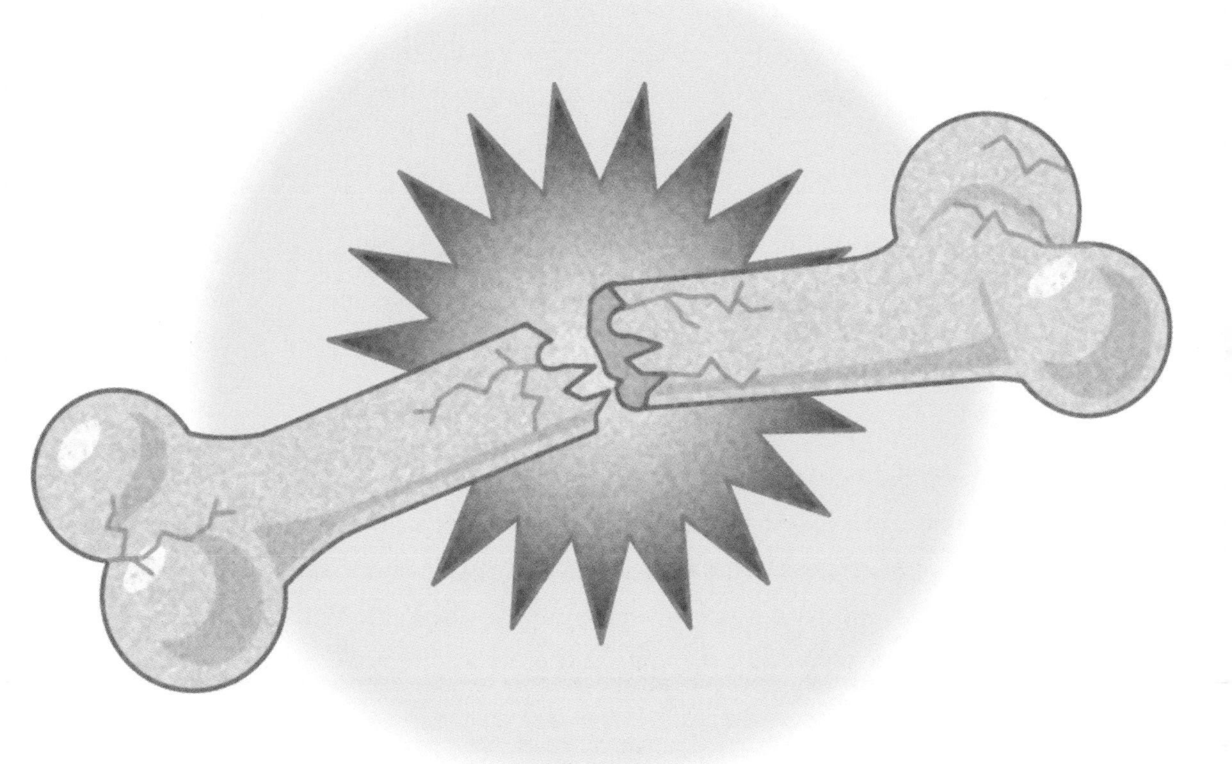

P is for PESTICIDES & POLLUTION

The higher up one eats on the food chain, the more one consumes concentrated toxins from flesh and body fluids of animals. Eat one portion of broccoli or lettuce and you'll ingest one dose of pesticides and dioxins. Ingest body fluids from animals who eat thousands of doses, and you deliver these same concentrated residues of poisons to your own body.

"A 1988 FDA survey of milk samples from grocery stores in 10 cities found that 73% of the samples contained pesticide residues."

Environmental Contamination and Toxicology, 1991; 47

"The lipophilic nature of dioxins results in higher concentrations in the fat of animal and fish products, and their excretion via milk secretion in dairy cattle may result in relatively high concentrations of dioxin contamination."

Journal of Animal Science, 1998 Jan, 76:1

"Atrazine is used primarily as a weed killer in the production of feed corn. This highly toxic herbicide has been linked to many kinds of cancer, including cancer of the breast, ovaries, uterus, and testicles, as well as leukemia and lymphoma... According to farming averages and data supplied by the Vermont Department of Agriculture, Ben & Jerry's farmers now use thousands of pounds of carcinogenic atrazine every year."

Food and Water Journal, Summer, 1998

"Dioxins are the most deadly substances ever assembled by man...170,000 times as deadly as cyanide..."

United Press International, March 11, 1983.

"The largest contributors to daily intake of chlorinated insecticides are dairy products, meat, fish, and poultry."

Sandra Steingraber, Ph.D., Living Downstream

"The level of dioxin in a single serving of the Ben & Jerry's World's Best Vanilla Ice Cream tested was almost 200 times greater than the 'virtually safe [daily] dose' determined by the Environmental Protection Agency."

Steve Milloy, author of junkscience.com

(Milloy tested samples of ice cream for dioxins.)

"The only safe level of dioxin exposure is no exposure at all."

Ben & Jerry's promotional literature

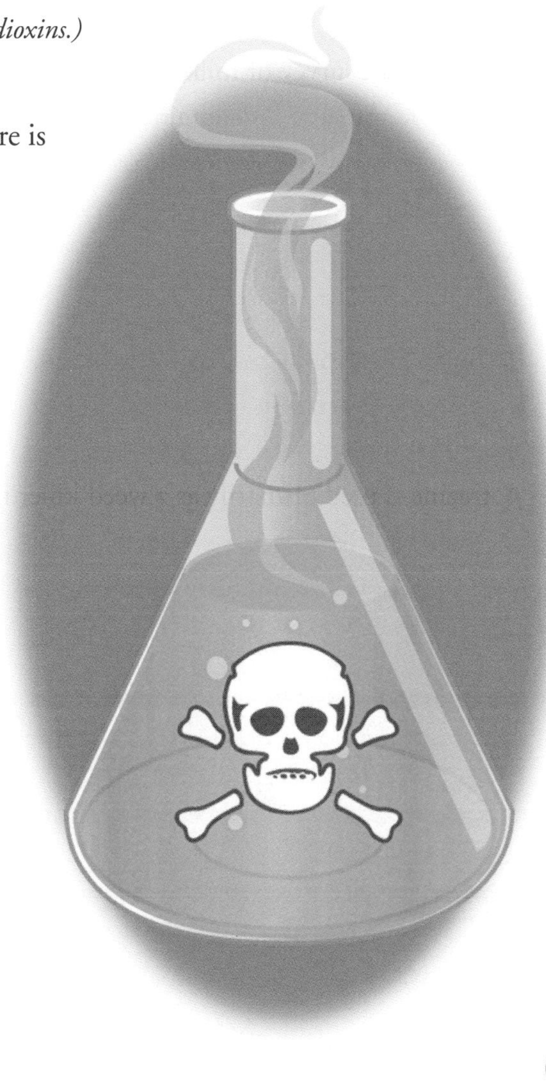

Q is for QUIXOTE SYNDROME

Don Quixote rode the Spanish countryside trying to fix the evils of the world by righting wrongs. He tilted at windmills and dreamed an impossible dream. So too do I dream an impossible dream. My "impossible dream" has become the dairy industry's nightmare. Here are some of the things people have said about my NOTMILK mission:

"If we required any reminder of the need to defend dairy products, we have received it in the person of Robert Cohen...Cohen has demonstrated an ability to take his allegations and spread them to the public through the Internet and through appearances on local radio and television programs."

Hoard's Dairyman, September 10, 1998

"Is Robert Cohen an enigma? Maybe. What's important is that he knows his enemy well - far better than we know ourselves. I have two lasting impressions. One is that underestimating Robert Cohen's ability to damage the dairy industry is a big mistake. The other is a profound wish that the man was on our side."

American Dairy Farmer Magazine, 10/1998, (Teresa Von Wagner editorial)

"The colorful NotMilk.com site delights in describing milk as a glass of 'pus with hormones and glue.' Its creator, Robert Cohen, who calls himself the Not Milk Man, keeps a list of diseases on the site that he believes are caused by milk."

New York Times Magazine Section, Sunday, December 24, 2000

"I joined Robert Cohen as a board member of his newly formed Dairy Education Board. I strongly recommend that you get more information on the dangers of dairy products by reading Cohen's book, available from the Dairy Education Board, 1-888-NOTMILK (888-668-6455), www.notmilk.com."

Julian Whitaker, M.D., Health & Healing, October 1998, Vol. 8, No. 10

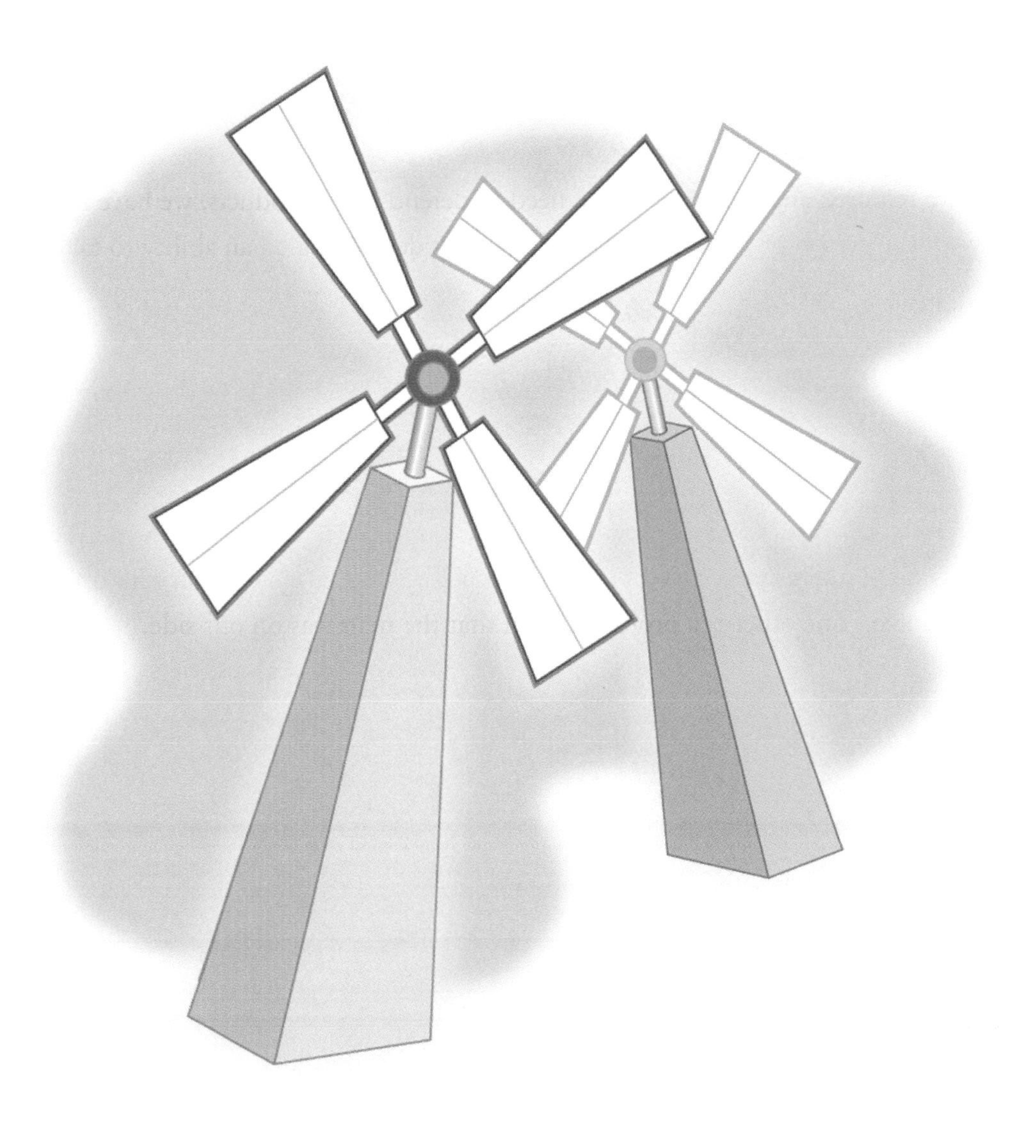

R is for RHEUMATOID ARTHRITIS

"Rheumatoid arthritis is more severe than osteoarthritis, is most common in the hands and feet, and is characterized by swelling of joints. Since this type of joint pain can be a symptom of a food allergy, dietary change sometimes has a profound effect. Dairy products, the most common food allergen, are one likely candidate as a contributing causative factor."

George Eisman, M.A., M.Sc., R.D., Vegetarian and Vegan Nutrition

"In the case of the eight-year-old female subject, juvenile rheumatoid arthritis was a milk allergy. After avoiding dairy products, all pain was gone in three weeks."

Journal of the Royal Society of Medicine, 1985, 78

"In 1964, I learned of the experiences of Dr. William Deamer of San Francisco. He had pointed out the frequency of milk protein's casual relationship to musculoskeletal pain in children and especially the so-called 'growing pains.' Since that time, I have had several children with what appeared to be early rheumatoid arthritis relieved and returned to good health by little more than reassurance and careful dietary manipulation."

Frank Oski, M.D., Don't Drink Your Milk

"Controlled trial of fasting and a one-year vegetarian diet eased symptoms of rheumatoid arthritis."

The Lancet, 1991, 338

"There is a colossal amount of information linking the consumption of milk to arthritis...and a multitude of other problems as documented by Hannah Allen,

Alec Burton, Viktoras Kulvinskas, F. M. Pottenger, Herbert M. Shelton, and N.L. Walker, among others."

Harvey and Marilyn Diamond, Fit for Life

"I once saw a 65-year-old man, Bob, who complained of neck stiffness and headaches. His hands were so stiff and sore. Bob lived to play golf. I instructed him to give up all milk and dairy products. Since giving up dairy products, he no longer experienced pain and headaches, and his hands were also pain-free. Joy, a 42-year-old woman noticed that her knees were pain-free after eliminating dairy products. Once, after drinking a glass of milk, her knees swelled within 20 minutes."

Daniel Twogood, D.C., No Milk

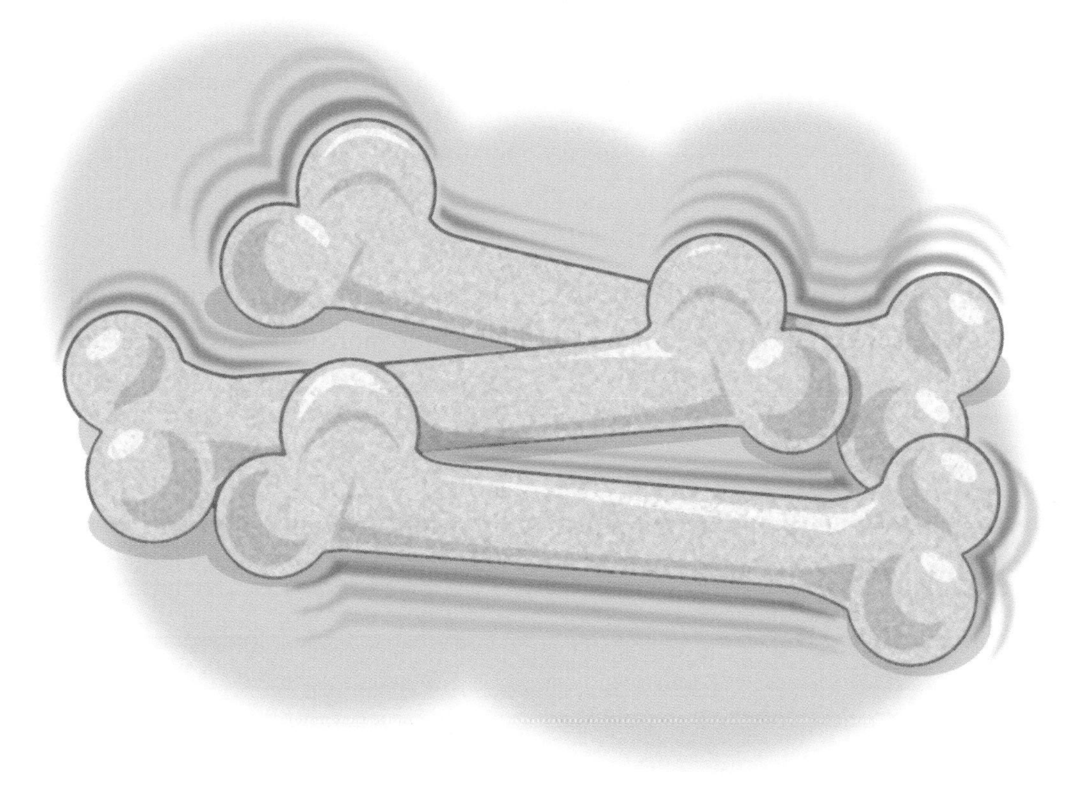

S is for SUDDEN INFANT DEATH

There are hundreds of scientific studies in the medical literature attesting to the fact that infants who are breast-fed have lower rates of sudden infant death syndrome (SIDS). Those performing the research rarely consider the alternative. Is it a component in breast milk that protects infants, or a component in the alternative (cow's milk protein) that triggers the allergic reaction? Cow's milk proteins are allergenic, and for some, the response is anaphylactic. Bronchioles fill with mucous, and some infants die.

"Breast feeding is known to protect an infant against gastrointestinal pathogens and epidemiological studies indicate that compared to breast-fed infants, formula-fed infants are at a greater risk of dying from sudden infant death syndrome."

Immunology & Medical Microbiology, 1999 Aug, 25:1-2

"Those infants who died of SIDS expressed inappropriate or inflammatory responses suggesting violent allergic reactions to a foreign protein. Lung tissue and cells showed responses similar to bronchial wall inflammation in asthma."

The Lancet, vol. 343, June 4, 1994

"Diet has a significant effect on the developing immune system...formula-fed babies, at the age of 3 months, were secreting low levels of serum antibodies to cow milk antigens contained in their formula."

Pediatric Allergy Immunology, August, 1994, 5(3)

"Those who consumed cow's milk were fourteen times more likely to die from diarrhea-related complications and four times more likely to die of pneumonia than were breast-fed babies. Intolerance and allergy to cow's milk products is a factor in sudden infant death syndrome."

The Lancet, vol. 344, November 5, 1994

"Hypersensitivity to milk is implicated as a cause of sudden death in infancy."

The Lancet, vol. 2, 7160, November 19, 1960

"Formula-fed infants developed symptoms of allergic rejection to cow milk proteins before one month of age. The recommended therapy is to avoid cow's milk."

PediatricAllergy-Immunology, 1994, 5(5 Supplement)

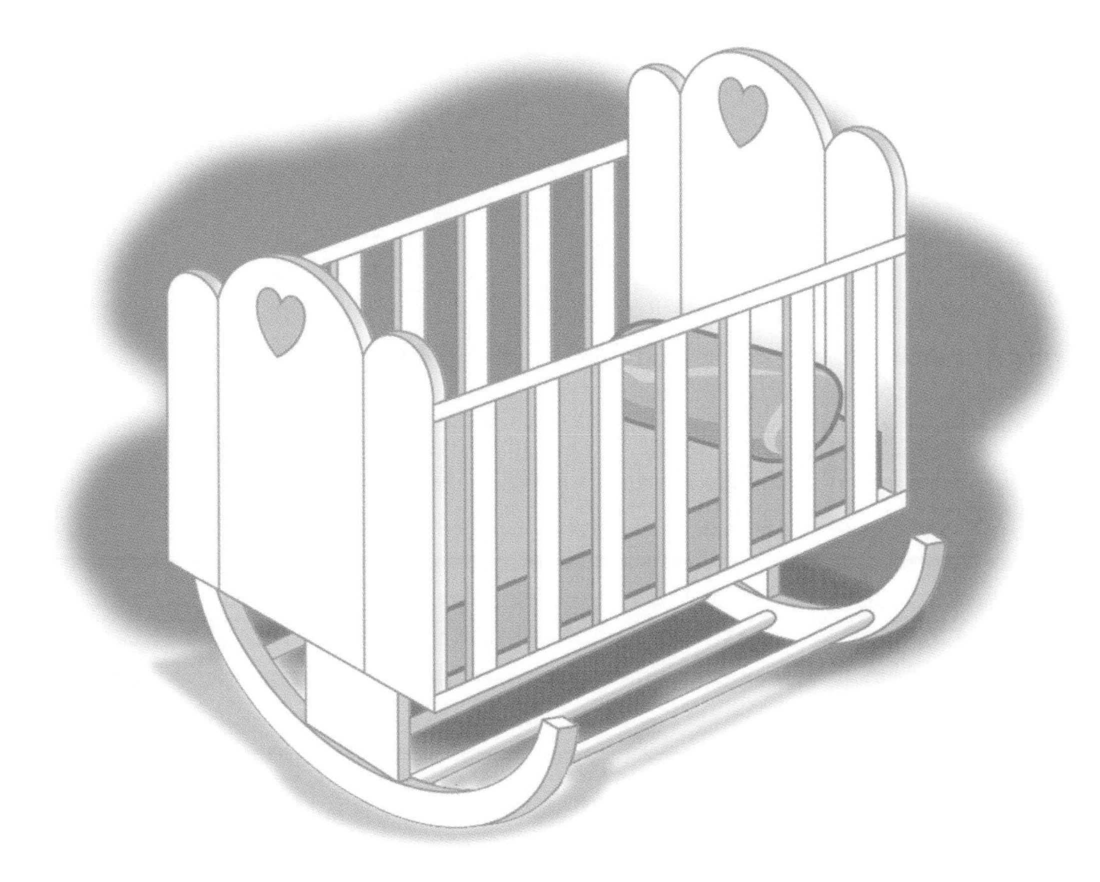

T is for TUBERCULOSIS

Russian Roulette is the most dangerous of games. Is one bullet in the chamber or five? Too many pasteurization errors have occurred in the past, and more will occur in the future. In 1985, 150,000 people got salmonella poisoning because milk was not pasteurized correctly in Chicago. Four people died. Nobody charted epidemiological data for subsequent tuberculosis death rates. Many of America's dairy cows are infected with tuberculosis. Does raw milk sound appetizing? Can you rely upon milk processors to properly pasteurize milk? Last year, there were dozens of major cheese recalls. Hundreds of thousands of cases of spoiled dairy products contained lethal virus and bacteria. Ingesting body fluids from diseased animals is a dangerous game of Russian Roulette.

As you review the first citation, ask yourself this question. Why does USDA allow milk from tuberculosis-infected herds to be sold?

"Mycobacterium bovis-infected dairy herd of 369 Holstein cows with lactation duration between 200 and 360 days was tested...170 cows had positive tuberculin test results, and 199 had negative results. Cows with positive test results produced less milk than did cows with negative test results. In this herd, tuberculosis was associated with a 4% decrease in milk production."

Journal of the American Veterinarian Association, 1998 Sep., 213:6

"Researchers and regulatory authorities were meeting to halt the rise and spread of tuberculosis from cows to humans, and to bring incidence to eradication levels."

Hoard's Dairyman, March 10, 1959

"Many diseases such as tuberculosis are transmissible by milk products."
Journal of Dairy Science, 1988; 71

"Some strains of mycobacteria, similar to those that are associated with tuberculosis, have been found to survive pasteurization."
The National Mastitis Council, Inc., 1970, Washington, D.C.

"A cow with pulmonary tuberculosis may swallow her own saliva and this, with the infected material coughed up from the lungs, then passes through the whole digestive tract, and remains as an active form of infection. Particles of infected dust or manure may contaminate the milk, or it may be infected directly from the tubercular udder."
Lincoln Lampert, Modern Dairy Products

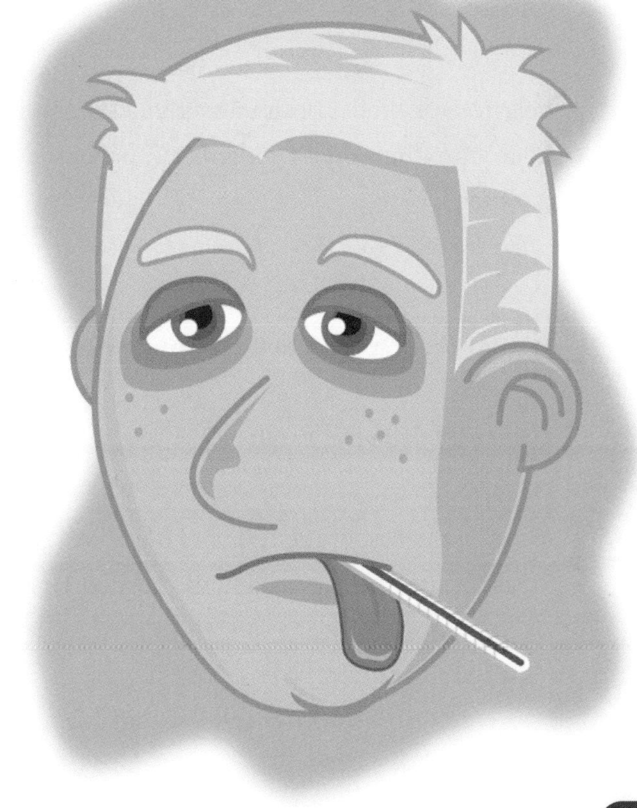

U is for UTERINE CANCER

Women between the ages of 25 and 65 have been successfully targeted by the marketing agents of the dairy industry's milk promotion board. What the dairy industry neglects to advertise is the fact that cow's milk contains a very powerful growth hormone, insulin-like growth factor-I (IGF-I). IGF-I is identical in humans and cows, and this hormone has been identified as a key factor in tumor growth.

"The uterus and ovary, like the breast, are hormone-sensitive organs. Not surprisingly, uterine and ovarian cancers are both linked to fatty diets in epidemiologic studies."

Cancer, 1966; 19

"Galactose is linked both to ovarian cancer and infertility. Women who consume dairy products on a regular basis, have triple the risk of ovarian cancer than other women."

The Lancet, 1989; 2

"Poor absorption of lactose may more than double the risk of ovarian cancer in women."

American Journal of Epidemiology, 1999; 150

"Interest in the role of the IGF axis in growth control and carcinogenesis has recently been increased by the finding of elevated serum (IGF-I) levels in association with three of the most prevalent cancers in the United States: prostate cancer, colorectal cancer, and lung cancer. IGFs serve as endocrine, autocrine, and paracrine stimulators of mitogenesis, survival, and cellular transformation."

Journal of Cellular Physiology, 2000 April, 183:1

"IGF-I reacts in a synergistic manner with estrogen, and plays a role in the growth and proliferation of ovarian cancer."

Journal of Clinical Endocrinology and Metabolism, Feb. 1994, 78(2)

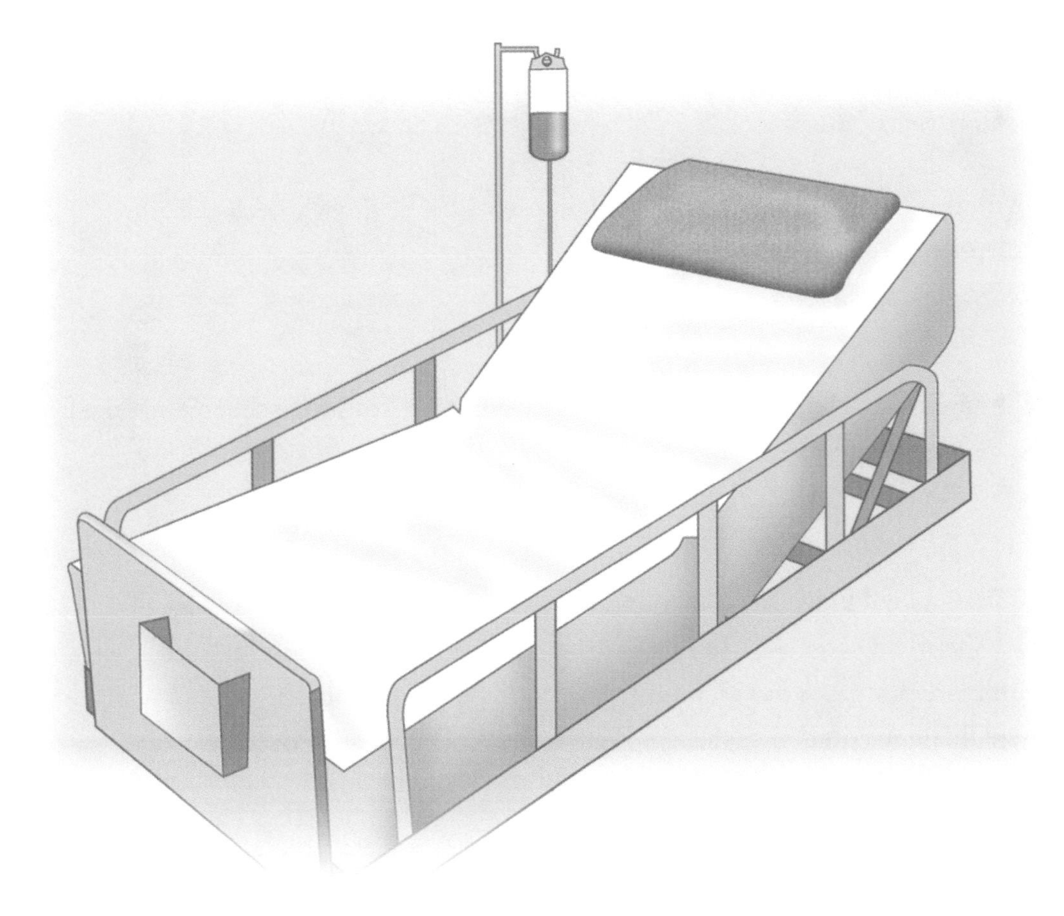

V is for VITAMIN D-EFICIENCY

How soon we forget! Children are taught in first grade that Vitamin D is the "sunshine vitamin." Vitamin D is a steroid hormone and is synthesized in one's body after skin is exposed to sunlight. Once the body has made enough, it will produce no more. Too much Vitamin D can be toxic and lead to bone loss.

"Exposure to sunlight provides most humans with their vitamin D requirement."
Journal of Nutrition, 1996; 126 (4, Supplement)

"Adults need 10-15 minutes of sunlight, two or three times a week to ensure proper Vitamin D levels."
Journal of Pediatrics, 1985; 107 (3)

"Consuming as little as 45 micrograms of Vitamin D-3 in young children has resulted in signs of overdose."
Pediatrics, 1963; 31

"Testing of 42 milk samples found only 12% within the expected range of Vitamin D content. Testing of 10 samples of infant formula revealed seven with more that twice the Vitamin D content reported on the label, one of which had more than four times the label amount. Vitamin D is toxic in overdose."
New England Journal of Medicine, 1992, 326

"Vitamin D increases aluminum absorption, and high aluminum levels in the body may cause an Alzheimer's-like disease."
Canadian Medical Association Journal, 1992 147(9)

"It has since been discovered that the Vitamin D necessary to absorb the calcium moving down the intestine must already have been in the bloodstream for a while; what is present with that calcium (in milk) is useless at that stage. Vitamin D is part of the mechanism to break bone down so that it can then stretch and grow. Thus an overdose of D can eventually lead to osteoporosis."

George Eisman, M.A., M.Sc., R.D., Vegetarian and Vegan Nutrition

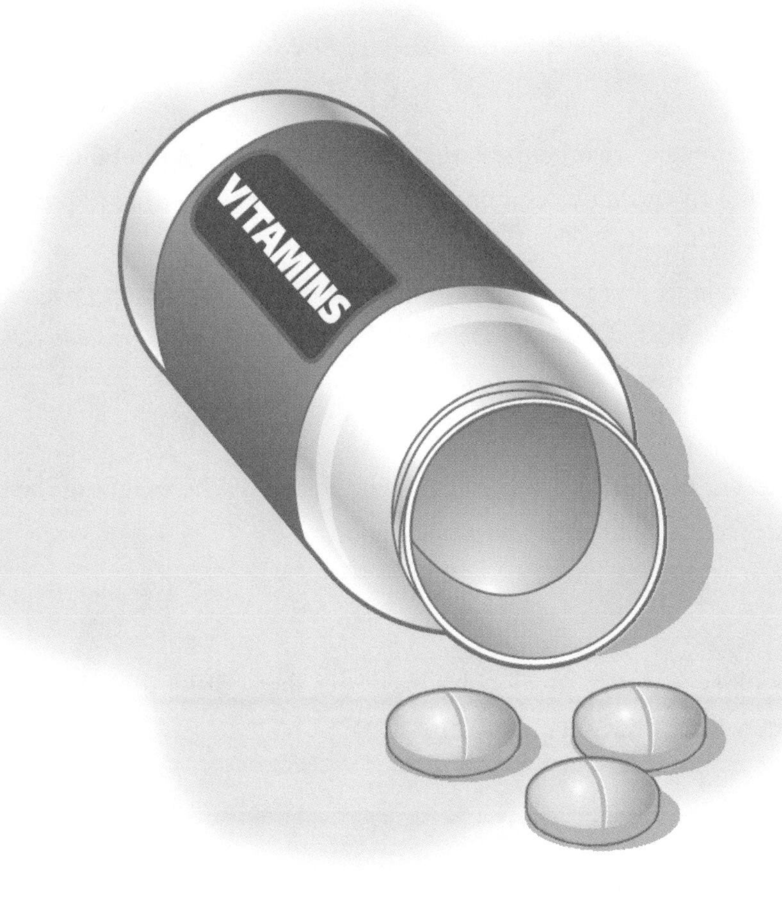

W is for WISCOWSINITIS

Some people call it "Cheesehead Syndrome.

"I have run into patients who undergo marked alterations in behavior patterns when ingesting dairy products, and whose behavior is totally changed by withholding them."

John J. Murray, M.D., Pediatrics (letter), 1979; 64(5)

"These dairymen are organized, they're adamant, they're militant, and they're massing an enormous amount of money that they're going to put into political activities, very frankly."

Secretary of the Treasury John Connally to President Richard Nixon, from the Watergate Tapes, March 23, 1971 (after President Nixon had received a $3 million cash gift from dairy industry representatives in the Oval Office).

"So don't drink milk for health. I am convinced on the weight of the scientific evidence that it does not do a body good."

Robert M. Kradjian, M.D., Save Yourself From Breast Cancer

"My illness is due to my doctor's insistence that I drink milk, a whitish fluid they force down helpless babies."

W.C. Fields

"Cow's milk in the past has been oversold as the perfect food, but we are now seeing that it isn't the perfect food at all and the government really shouldn't be behind any efforts to promote it as such."

Benjamin Spock, M.D., Los Angeles Times, November 18, 1992

"I would call milk perhaps the most unhealthful vehicle for calcium that one could possibly imagine, which is the only thing people really drink it for, but whenever you challenge existing dogma...people are resistant."

Neal Barnard, M.D., Director of the Physician's Committee for Responsible Medicine
www.pcrm.org

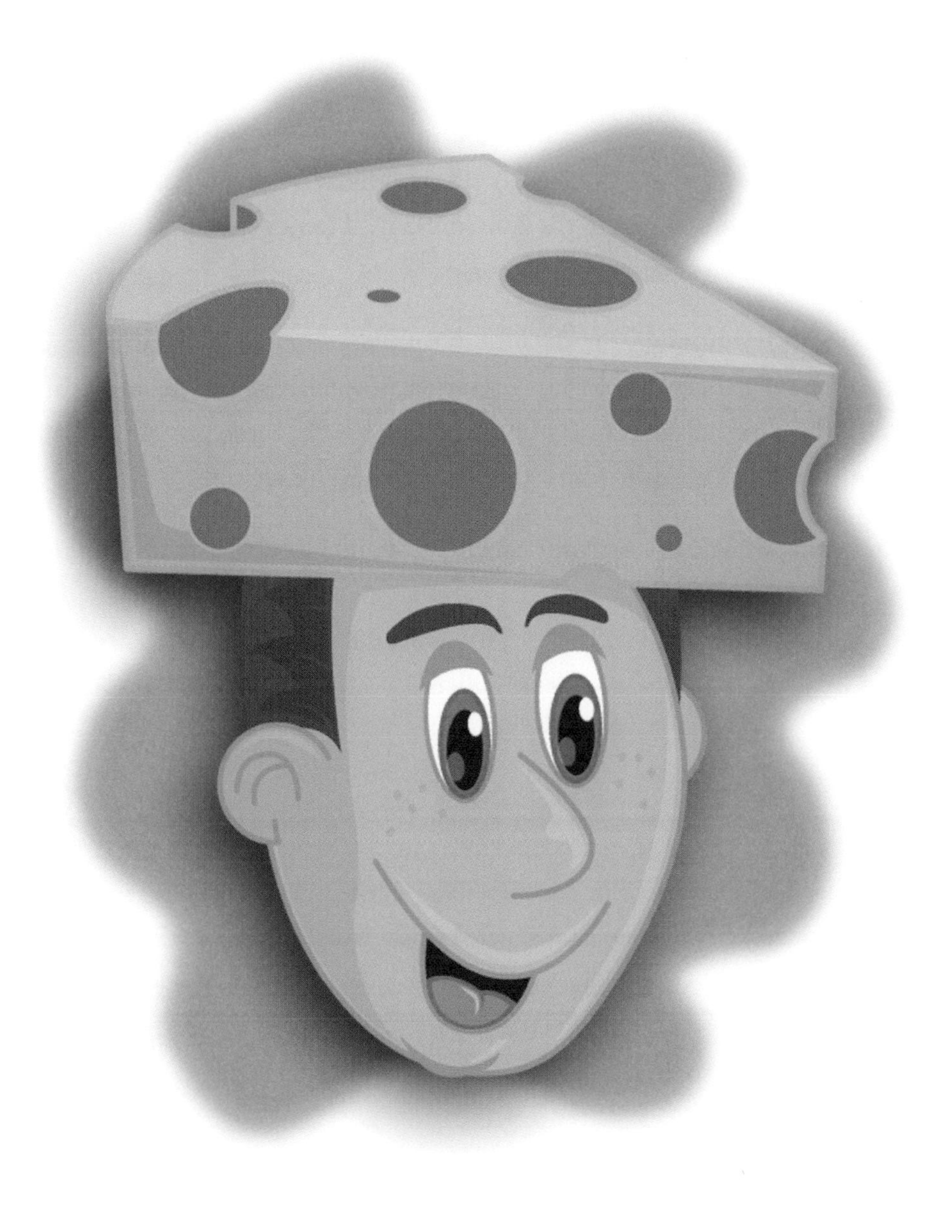

X is for XANTHENE OXIDASE

WHAT IS HOMOGENIZATION? When milk is passed through a fine filter at pressures equal to 4,000 pounds per square inch, the fat globules (liposomes) are made smaller (micronized) by a factor of 10 times or more. These molecules become evenly dispersed within the liquid milk.

Milk is a hormonal delivery system. With homogenization, milk becomes a very powerful and efficient way of bypassing normal digestive processes and delivering steroid and protein hormones to the human body. Homogenization is technology's way of improving upon nature's mechanism.

Through homogenization, fat molecules in milk become smaller and become "capsules" for substances that bypass digestion. Proteins would normally be digested in the stomach or gut. By homogenizing milk, these proteins are not broken down and are absorbed into the bloodstream intact.

Two Connecticut researchers, Oster and Ross, demonstrated that cow proteins survive digestion. Their heart patients developed antibodies to bovine proteins after consuming homogenized milk. This proved that milk proteins are not destroyed by digestion. Hormones in milk are protected, survive digestion, and exert powerful effects on the human body.

Science teaches that the survival of protein hormones after ingestion is not possible because of the strength of stomach acid and enzymatic activity. Oster and Ross pointed a finger of blame at the homogenization process. They discovered the presence of an enzyme, bovine xanthene oxidase (XO), which, in theory, should not have survived digestion. The XO Factor was identified as the element that destroyed one-third of the cellular material in atrial cells of heart attack victims during their five-year study.

"Atherosclerotic patients exhibit an immune response to bovine xanthene oxidase."

American Laboratory, August 1974

"Milk antibodies are significantly elevated in the blood of patients with heart disease."

Proceedings of the Society for Experimental Biology & Medicine, 1981: 163

"Bovine milk xanthene oxidase (BMXO) may be absorbed and may enter the cardiovascular system. BMXO antibodies are found in greater quantities in those patients who consume the largest volumes of homogenized milk and milk products."

Kurt Oster, M.D., and Donald Ross, Ph.D., The X-O Factor

"Seventy-three out of the 94 people tested (of all ages) had antibodies to XO."

Proceedings of the Society of Experimental Biology & Medicine, 1979;160

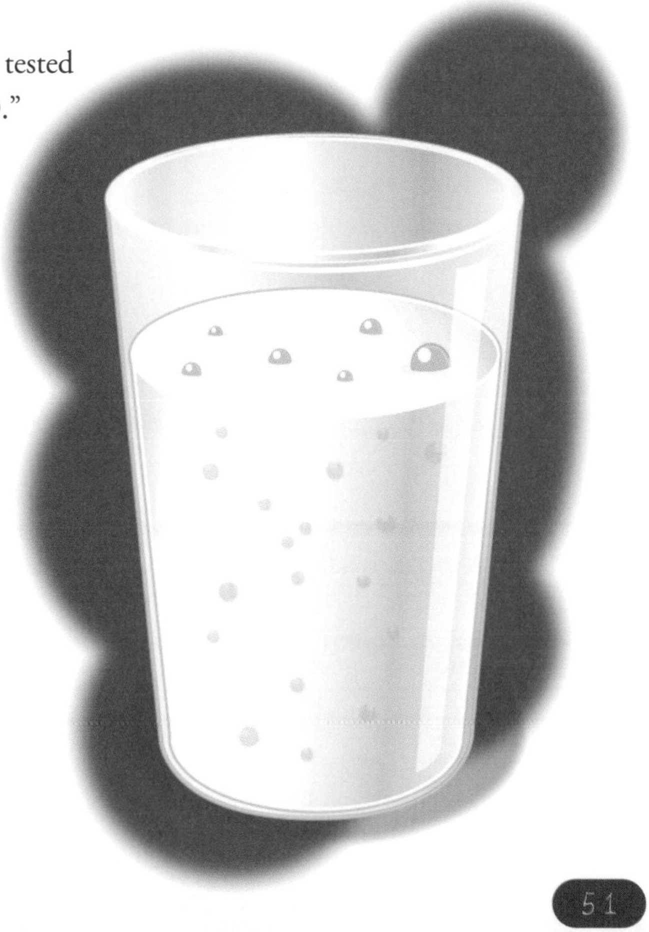

Y is for YIN/YANG

Yin and Yang are spiritual forces in Chinese philosophy. Together they form the life-giving power of the universe, but apart they are opposite sides of the pole. Yin is the moon; the soft, the feminine, the receptive and even side of things. Yang is the sun; the bright and powerful masculine force, the odd and wild side. Vegetarians drink milk and eat dairy products. Vegans eat no animal products. Meat eaters and vegetarians are the Yang. By eating animal flesh or drinking their body fluids, one ingests their hormones. Vegans eat no animal hormones. Vegans are the Yin.

"Scientific data suggest positive relationships between a vegetarian diet and reduced risk for several chronic degenerative diseases and conditions, including obesity, coronary artery disease, hypertension, diabetes mellitus, and some types of cancer."

Journal of the American Dietetic Association, November 1997, 97(1)

"Atherosclerosis is rare in peoples whose diet over the life span is predominantly vegetarian and low in calories, total lipids, saturated lipids and cholesterol."

Louis Katz, Nutrition and Atherosclerosis, 1958

"Vegan diets can meet the nutrient and energy needs of pregnant women."

Pediatrics, 1989; 84

"Reduced colorectal cancer risk is associated with increased consumption of fiber, vegetables, and fruit."

Cancer Cause Control, 1991; 1

"Vegetarians often have lower mortality rates from several chronic degenerative diseases than do nonvegetarians."

British Medical Journal, 1996; 313

"Vegetarian diets low in fat or saturated fat have been used successfully as part of comprehensive health programs to reverse severe coronary artery disease."

Journal of the American Medical Association, 1995; 274

"Incidence of lung and colorectal cancer is lower in vegetarians than in nonvegetarians."

American Journal of Clinical Nutrition, 1994; 59 (supplement)

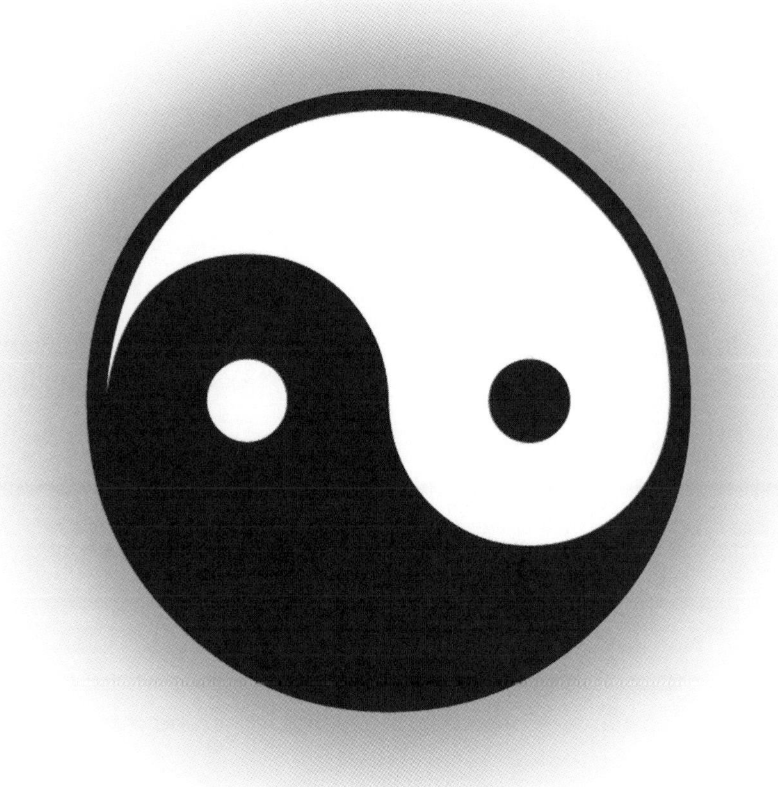

Z is for ZITS

Acne occurs when steroids (androgens) stimulate the sebaceous glands within the skin's hair follicles. These glands then secrete an oily substance called sebum. When sebum, bacteria and dead skin cells build up on your skin, the pores become blocked, creating a zit.

What do you expect? When teenagers combine their own surging hormones with dietary saturated animal fat, cholesterol, steroid hormones, dead white blood cells, and cow pus, they're gonna get zits. The good news...The cure is an easy one: NOTMILK!

"As pointed out by Dr. Jerome Fisher, 'About 80 percent of cows that are giving milk are pregnant and are throwing off hormones continuously.' Progesterone breaks down into androgens, which have been implicated as a factor in the development of acne...Dr. Fisher observed that his teenage acne patients improved as soon as the milk drinking stopped."

Frank Oski, M.D., Don't Drink Your Milk

"We studied the effects of growth hormone (GH) and insulin-like growth factors (IGFs), alone and with androgen, on sebaceous epithelial cell growth...IGF-I was the most potent stimulus of DNA synthesis. These data are consistent with the concept that increases in GH and IGF production contribute in complementary ways to the increase in sebum production during puberty."

Endocrinology, 1999 Sep, 140:9

"Acne usually begins at puberty, when an increase in androgens causes an increase in the size and activity of pilosebaceous glands. If a food is suspected, it should be omitted for several weeks and then eaten in substantial quantities to determine if acne worsens."

MERCK Manual, Merck & Company, 2000

"Acne is an end-organ hyper-response to androgens...These data show that sebaceous glands are stimulated by androgens to varying degrees and support the theory of an end-organ response in acne."

British Journal of Dermatology, 1998 July, 139:1

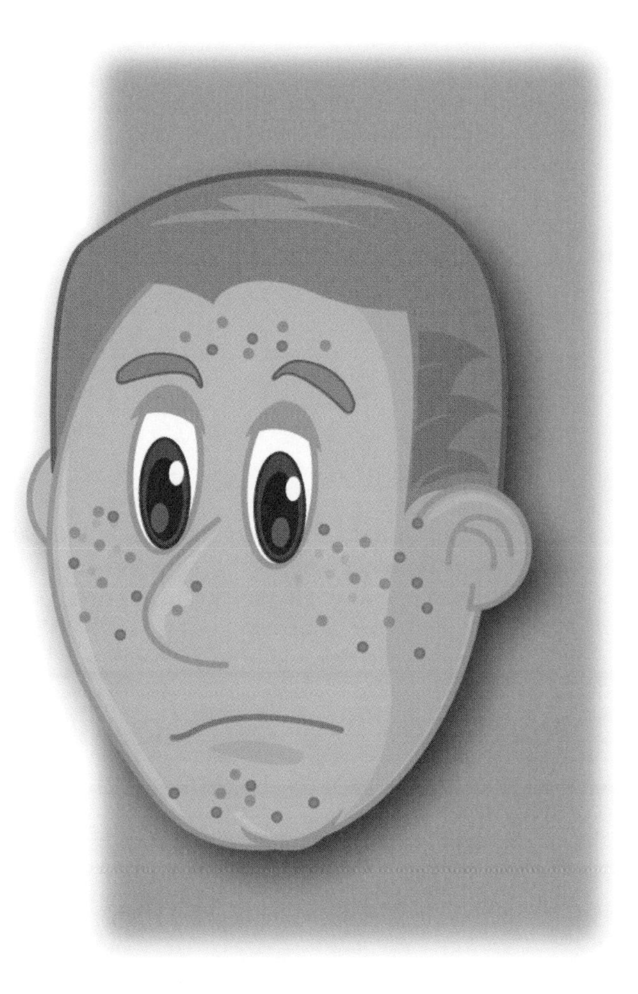

Final Exam (Multiple Choice)

1) The *Townsend Medical Letter for Doctors* said this about cow's milk:

a) Adult humans require cow's milk for optimum health. Adult cows need human milk for optimum health. Adult dogs should drink pig's milk for optimum health. Adult pigs require aardvark milk for optimum health.

b) Cream cheese has been shown to be an effective decay preventative dentifrice that can be of significant value when used in a conscientiously applied program of oral hygiene and regular professional care.

c) Cow's milk hormones, saturated fat, and cholesterol offer enormous benefit for young children. A diet of concentrated milk products (cheese, ice cream, and butter) will insure that our subscriber base remains healthy, as will the future cash flow of physicians who read this newsletter.

d) Cow's milk has been linked to a variety of health problems, including: mucous production, hemoglobin loss, childhood diabetes, heart disease, athersclerosis, arthritis, kidney stones, mood swings, depression, irritability, and allergies.

2) The most powerful growth hormone produced in a cow's body (and found in cow's milk) is identical to the most powerful growth hormone in the human body. That hormone is called IGF. IGF stands for:

a) I've Got Flatulence

b) Idiots Grow Fat

c) Icelandic Gouda's Fabulous

d) Insulin-like Growth Factor

3) The *Lancet, Journal of Cellular Physiology*, and *European Journal of Cancer* have all identified IGF as:

a) A food supplement that removes wrinkles, freckles, cellulite, zits, and elevates I.Q. points.

b) The most powerful aphrodisiac found in food.

c) The thick mucous-like substance in cow's milk proteins responsible for the profitability of the Charmin toilet paper company.

d) The key factor in the growth and proliferation of breast, prostate, and lung cancers.

4) At the first sign of heat treatment (pasteurization), many bacteria in milk:

a) Begin a mating ritual that embarrasses even the most permissively liberal of microbiologists.

b) Begin to gag, then lose the contents of their tiny bacterial pouches, secreting their body wastes and toxins into the milk.

c) Perspire nano-liters of sweat before dying, their lifeless bodies drowning and adding subtle flavors to the milk.

d) Form spores. Spore is a Greek word for seed. When the milk cools, spores re-emerge into their original bacterial forms.

5) Mycobacterium Paratuberculosis is:

a) The name of the Serbian general turned priest who won the 2001 Nobel Peace Prize by writing, "When NATO Bombs Drop, Forget the Child, Save the Cow."

b) Something that your mate will not believe you caught from a toilet seat in a public restroom.

c) The polite thing to say to a Flemish dairy farmer who sneezes liters of phlegm.

d) A bacterium found in many of America's dairy herds and 100% of Crohn's disease patients. These bacteria are not destroyed by pasteurization, and cross the species barrier from cow to human.

6) A leading diabetes journal (*Diabetes Care*) wrote the following in 1974: "More than 20 well-documented studies have prompted one researcher to say the link between milk and juvenile diabetes is "very solid." The dairy industry's response was to:

a) Design a chocolate milk mustache advertisement that used the Rugrats, children's cartoon characters, to promote milk drinking for infants.

b) Design milk ads using Pokemon characters and Kermit the Frog to promote the consumption of milk for young children.

c) Neither A nor B

d) Both A and B

7) The Chief of Pediatrics at Johns Hopkins Medical School (Frank Oski) and America's most famous pediatrician, Benjamin Spock, agreed upon this therapy for ear infections:

a) Both physicians studied at the French Institute of Van Goghzia, and agreed that surgical removal of the ear would effectively eliminate ear infections.

b) Both physicians recommended that surgical implants be considered for children suffering from ear infections.

c) Both physicians agreed that ritalin, valium, and a continuous diet of Benadryl and other antihistamines would be an appropriate therapy to treat chronic ear infections.

d) Both physicians recommended a protocol in which all milk and dairy products should be eliminated from the diets of all children.

8) Saturated bovine fat contained in milk, cheese, ice cream and other dairy products:

a) Is necessary for human brain development, cognitive functioning, and become precursors for neural transmitting substances.

b) Is a vital component of human synnovial fluid that lubricates the joints.

c) Have been identified as the key factors in "getting the juices going."

d) Have been identified as the single-most causative factor of America's obesity epidemic, and the link to heart disease being America's number-one killer.

9) Cows treated with the genetically engineered bovine growth hormones produce milk that has been proven to:

a) Result in more snaps, crackles, and pops per standard bowl of Rice Krispies.

b) Be identical to naturally occurring milk.

c) Promote weight loss, reduce flatulence, and eliminate cellulite.

d) Result in an increase of insulin-like growth factor, a hormone identified as the key role player in fueling the growth of human breast cancer, prostate cancer, lung cancer, and colon cancer.

10) An epidemiological study of mortality rates in 24 nations found that consumption of these foods resulted in the highest correlation coefficient to heart disease:

a) Fresh vegetables, particularly broccoli and rutabaga.
b) Beans, beans, NOT good for the hearty, the more you eat, the worse for the artery.
c) Whole wheat berries and barley (these large uncooked grains get stuck in arteries causing coronary thrombosis.)
d) Milk and dairy products.

11) The *Journal of Pediatrics* revealed that cow's milk proteins can cause blood loss from the intestinal tract, reduce the body's supply of iron, and cause anemia. The recommended therapy:

a) Add powdered iron filings to your next bowl of cereal with soy milk.
b) Bite the bullet.
c) Drink a twelve-ounce glass of human breast milk with your cookies.
d) Avoid all cow milk and dairy products.

12) According to the *New England Journal of Medicine*, "Chronic diarrhea is the most common gastrointestinal symptom of intolerance of cow's milk among children." As a parent, what is the best method of eliminating this messy problem?

a) Eliminate the source. Sell your children to the next band of slave traders moving through your neighborhood.
b) Save cork stoppers from champagne bottles, and use 'em when they're needed!
c) When the condition occurs, add one cup of corn starch to three tablespoons of prune juice, stir well, and use a number seven syringe to inject the paste directly into your child's stomach cavity.
d) Eliminate all milk and dairy products from your child's diet.

13) Should milk consumers worry about harmful bacterial infections resulting from milk and dairy consumption? Which statement(s) is/are true?

a) According to the *Journal of Dairy Science*, butter readily supports growth of salmonella at room temperature, but refrigeration or freezing for brief periods does not eliminate it. Salmonella can remain viable in butter for up to 9 months.
b) According to the *New England Journal of Medicine*, listeria organisms excreted in cow's milk escape pasteurization, grow well at refrigerator temperatures, and are ingested by consumers.
c) According to leading food journals, curing alone may not be a sufficient pathogen control step to eliminate salmonella, listeria, and E. coli from cheese. A drop of sour milk may contain more than 50 million bacteria.
d) All of the above.

14) Lactose intolerance affects 75% of the world's population. Symptoms include bloating, flatulence, abdominal pain, and diarrhea. The cure for eliminating lactose intolerance:

a) Having elective stomach-staple surgery, tying off your intestines, and satisfying future nutritional needs by intravenous feeding.
b) Investing your assets in a portfolio that includes the Pampers diaper company and Johnson's baby powder, buying a year's supply of adult stay-dries, and drinking all the milk you want.
c) Taking an antidote, lactaid, so that you may tolerate the poison, milk.
d) Don't drink your milk.

15) Normal cows become Mad Cows after:

a) Their mothers force them to drink three glasses of human breast milk each day.
b) They witness their mothers and sisters being loaded onto packed trucks and shipped to slaughterhouses.
c) They are injected with genetically engineered hormones that swell their udders to painful proportions which require three milkings per day.
d) They are fed blood meal, bone meal, and flesh from their relatives.

16) Nutritionists agree: Humans need to eat protein. Eighty percent of milk protein is 'CASEIN.' When casein is isolated from milk, it can be used:

a) In the manufacturing process for plastic.
b) As a glue to hold together wood in furniture.
c) As an adhesive to attach a label to a beer bottle.
d) All of the above.

17) Read the following statements carefully. Which ONE is NOT true?

a) Countries with the highest rates of osteoporosis, such as the United States, England, and Sweden, consume the most milk. China and Japan, where people eat much less protein and dairy food, have low rates of osteoporosis.
b) Osteoporosis is caused by a number of things, one of the most important being too much dietary protein. Dietary protein increases production of acid in the blood which is neutralized by calcium mobilized from the skeleton. Increasing one's protein intake by 100% may cause calcium loss to double.
c) Data from the 12-year Harvard study of 78,000 women indicate that women consuming greater amounts of calcium from dairy foods had significantly increased risks of hip fractures, while no increase in fracture risk was observed for the same levels of calcium from nondairy sources.
d) American women have been consuming an average of two pounds of milk per day for their entire lives, yet thirty million American women have osteoporosis. Therefore, drinking milk prevents bone loss.

18) The level of dioxin in a single serving of the Ben & Jerry's World's Best Vanilla Ice Cream tested was almost 200 times greater than the safe daily dose determined by the Environmental Protection Agency. What did Ben Cohen of Ben & Jerry's fame have to say regarding dioxins?

a) "Our containers are environmentally friendly, and dioxin-free, so just dump the ice cream, and eat the container."
b) "I just had quadruple bypass heart surgery. Please put your question in writing, and I'll have my staff get back to you."
c) "We never realized you'd be supremely nuts to continue eating our Natural Nutty-Nuts Supreme Surprise."
d) (Before the test): "The only safe level of dioxin exposure is no exposure at all." (After the test): "It's in the environment."

19) Do pesticides end up in milk, cheese, and butter? Which one of the following statements is NOT accurate?

a) A 1988 FDA survey of milk samples from grocery stores in 10 cities found that 73% of the samples contained pesticide residues.

b) More than 2,200 samples of cow's milk were tested in India, and 85% of the samples contained pesticides levels above human tolerance limits.

c) The pesticides chlordane and heptachlor cause cancer, harm the immune system and are endocrine disruptors. Dairy cattle in Oahu were fed pineapple leaves containing heptachlor residues. As a result, the local milk and dairy supply remained contaminated for years.

d) According to the National Fluid Milk Processors, no pesticide residues have ever been found in milk and dairy products.

20) Milk contains somatic cells, which are dead red and white blood cells. Another name for somatic cells is "pus cells." America's Food and Drug Administration sets the legal standard for the allowable number of pus cells that can be sold in milk. One liter of American milk may contain no more than:

a) 75 hundred pus cells

b) 75 thousand pus cells

c) 75 million pus cells

d) 750 million pus cells

21) Which of the following statements did NOT appear in the British medical journal *Lancet*?

a) Hypersensitivity to milk is implicated as a cause of sudden death in infancy.

b) Those infants who died of SIDS expressed inappropriate or inflammatory responses suggesting violent allergic reactions to a foreign protein. Lung tissue and cells showed responses similar to bronchial wall inflammation in asthma.

c) Those who consumed cow's milk were fourteen times more likely to die from diarrhea-related complications and four times more likely to die of pneumonia than were breast-fed babies. Intolerance and allergy to cow's milk products is a factor in sudden infant death syndrome.

d) Children under the age of two years who consume more that one-pint of fortified brandy before going to bed are prone to sudden infant death.

22) On March 23, 1971, Secretary of the Treasury John Connally said to President Richard Nixon (recorded on a Watergate tape): "These dairymen are organized, they're adamant, they're militant, and they're massing an enormous amount of money that they're going to put into political activities." Why did Connally make this statement?

a) Dairy reps had placed the severed head of a dairy cow in Nixon's bed, making him an offer he couldn't refuse.

b) Richard Nixon had just been presented with a compromising surveillance photo of JFK, RFK, and Marilyn Monroe sporting what appeared to be the dairy industry's first milk mustache ad.

c) President Nixon had just been given a $10 gift certificate to Dairy Queen from dairy industry representatives in the Oval Office.
d) President Nixon had just been given a $3 million cash gift from dairy industry representatives in the Oval Office.

23) Children are taught in first grade that Vitamin D is the "sunshine vitamin." Which statement about vitamin D is NOT true?

a) Adults need 10-15 minutes of sunlight, two or three times a week to ensure proper Vitamin D levels.
b) Vitamin D is toxic in overdose. Consuming as little as 45 micrograms of Vitamin D-3 in young children has resulted in signs of overdose. Testing of 10 samples of infant formula revealed seven with more that twice the Vitamin D content reported on the label, one of which had more than four times the label amount.
c) Vitamin D increases aluminum absorption, and high aluminum levels in the body may cause an Alzheimer's-like disease.
d) If boys and girls do not drink milk with Vitamin D added, when they turn 40, their bones will become brittle, and break, and they'll need hip replacement surgery.

24) What has NOT been identified as a cause of acne?

a) Acne occurs when steroids (androgens) stimulate the sebaceous glands within the skin's hair follicles. These glands then secrete an oily substance called sebum. When sebum, bacteria and dead skin cells build up on skin, the pores become blocked, creating acne.
b) About 80 percent of cows that are giving milk are pregnant and are throwing off hormones continuously. Progesterone breaks down into androgens, which have been implicated as a factor in the development of acne. Hormones found in cow's milk include: estradiol, estriol, progesterone, prolactin, and oxytocin.
c) The *Journal of Endocrinology* studied the effects of growth hormone (GH) and insulin-like growth factors (IGF-I), alone and with androgen, on sebaceous epithelial cell growth. IGF-I was the most potent stimulus of DNA synthesis, contributing to the increase in sebum production during puberty.
d) Acne is caused by frogs, sugar, snails, spice, puppy dog tails, and everything nice.

25) What is NOT true about the vegetarian NOTMILK lifestyle?

a) According to the *Journal of the American Dietetic Association*, there is a positive correlation between a vegetarian diet and reduced risk for obesity, coronary artery disease, hypertension, diabetes mellitus, and cancer."
b) According to the *British Medical Journal*, vegetarians often have lower mortality rates from several chronic degenerative diseases than do non-vegetarians. Significant athersclerosis is rare in peoples whose diet over the life span is predominantly vegetarian and low in calories, saturated fat, and cholesterol.
c) According to the *Journal of the American Medical Association*, vegetarian diets low in fat or saturated fat have been used successfully as part of comprehensive health programs to reverse severe coronary artery disease.
d) Vegans live an average of two decades less than meat-eaters and milk drinkers which is just fine with carnivores, who are saved from having to listen to twenty or more years of irritating lecturing, preaching, and bragging.

Score Your Test Results

Let's make this process really simple, shall we? D is the correct answer for all 25 multiple-choice questions. D as in "duh." This way, you won't have to scribble in the margins of this book as you scan back and forth between questions and answers. (Don't you just hate those tests where they put the answers upside down…in tiny print?) Unfortunately, there might be some of you who have been drinking cow's milk since childhood, so you still don't get it, and may never get it. Award yourself four points for each correct response.

1) d	8) d	15) d	22) d
2) d	9) d	16) d	23) d
3) d	10) d	17) d	24) d
4) d	11) d	18) d	25) d
5) d	12) d	19) d	
6) d	13) d	20) d	
7) d	14) d	21) d	

If you scored 88 or better, you are either a vegan (eat no animal flesh and drink no body fluids) or a professional cheesehead. You know milk issues like few people do. You are to be congratulated for your wisdom!

If you scored between 72 and 84, you haven't been paying attention to the real science contained in *MILK A-Z.* Go back and study!

If you scored between 52 and 68, you've passed...barely, but only because we're grading on a curve. Go sit by yourself in a quiet little corner and repeat over and over again the following mantra: "Pus with hormones and glue...pus with hormones and glue...pus with hormones and glue." Use this visualization the next time you are tempted to slurp ice cream, munch cheddar, or drown yourself in a tub of melted butter.

If you scored below the 50th percentile, instruct your attorney to re-write your last will and testament and leave your estate to your doctors. They'll ultimately end up with most of your money, anyway. Heart disease claims the lives of nearly two out of three Americans, and cancers account for one out of every three deaths. The average American spends ten years dying from coronary-related events or carcinomas. What you don't know about milk may kill you. The healthy alternative? Discover the fountain of youth: NOTMILK!

If you scored under 25, you've got very little hope remaining. You are an udderly absurd excuse for a human, and have earned the right to continue to consume body fluids from diseased animals. If you are still ambulatory, treat yourself to Domino's Pizza for dinner and slurp Ben and Jerry's Ice Cream for dessert. Set your alarm clock for a 12-hour wake up call. This might be your last chance, so pay attention to your body's signals. If your internal sludge and congestion do not convince you, nothing ever will.

Robert Cohen

www.notmilk.com

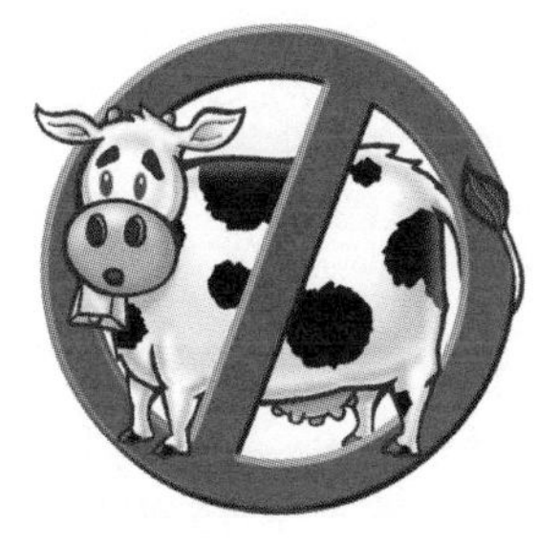